MUST WE GROW OLD

From Pauling to Prigogine to Toynbee

by

Daniel Hershey, Ph.D.

A Basal Book
1984

Published by
Basal Books
726 Lafayette Avenue
Cincinnati, Ohio 45220

A Division of Basal-Tech, Inc.

Copyright © 1984
Daniel Hershey

Library of Congress Catalog Card Number: 83-71510

All rights reserved. No part of this publication may be reproduced or transmitted in any form or by any means, electronic or mechanical, including photocopy, recording, or any information storage or retrieval system, without permission in writing from the publisher.

CONTENTS

CHAPTERS	PAGE
1. A Journey	1

(What happens to our souls when we die)

2. In God We Trust 3
(Life and death: from George, the carbon atom; to Mary, the smallpox virus; to Mark, the human; to Tiny Alice, who loved to play with her Milky Way)

3. Longevity: Theories and Speculation 15
(From ancient history to the present)

4. Death in Conclusion 46
(A father to his young son, on the meaning of death)

5. My Aged Father 52
(Retiring to oblivion)

6. Losses with Age 56
(What our old bodies can't do anymore)

7. Hey Michael, It's Your Daddy 62
(What an aging father feels while watching his son grow)

8. Neutralizing the Losses 68
(To slow the aging process)

9. Reflections in an Aging Eye 77
(The wear and tear of growing up in New York)

10. Mutations 86
(Dividing cells and what can go wrong)

11. Work 90
(It may cause aging)

12. Collagen: Stiff and Stiffer 93
(And slower and slower)

13. Lost Horizons 99
(Mrs. G. shouldn't have gone to that nursing home)

14. Nutrition Against Aging 103
(You are what you eat)

15. This You Never Learned in School 118
(Piquant lessons in growing up)

16. Energy, Entropy, Exercise, Basal Metabolism and Lifespan 125
(The driving forces of life)

17. The Aging Professor 202
(Becoming an old teacher)

18. Cities, Corporations, Civilizations: Size; Structure; Stability; Senescence 213
(Must they grow old. Why they die)

19. A Kid's View of Death 246
(An unreal event)

20. Do You Know Me, Michael? 247
(An aging father pleads for understanding)

21. The Challenge: The Search for Unifying Principles 248
(Finding order and disorder everywhere)

PROLOGUE

How old are you?
How do you know?
Who is older, you or I?
How old are your lungs? Your heart? Eyes? Skin? Hair?
There's a difference, you know.
And a variability to lifespan. Man versus woman, between animals, trees, corporations and civilizations.

Can you hear time flying? Listen to the silence. Do you hear the clock ticking away, tolling the beginning, the middle, and the end?

I know I am but an infinitesimal cog in a larger, infinite order of things. We shall be born, live and die, and in being, alter the universe. The march towards infinity will be affected ever so slightly by my record of existence. Very few will be aware of my history. But I know, and by knowing I endeavor to construct a meaningful record.

Daniel Hershey

Chapter 1

A Journey

I died last night and it was very interesting. Not nearly as bad as I thought it would be; quite a surprising experience you might say. It takes a moment of pain, pretty much like a pin prick, after the last breath, for our bodies to turn off all those intricately connected switches, sending a signal from the brain to all parts, that this is the end. First the brain dampens its buzzing circuits, then the heart ceases its contractions much as an engine grinds to a halt after the power is shut off and finally muscles, blood vessels, skin and bones relax. The word gets out to our red and white cells. The foreign bacteria and viruses who exist parasitically on and within us get the message. It's over; the system is inoperable. It's time to get out.

And I got out too. That's what I meant by this death experience being a surprising event. I never dreamed that there was more to me than skin and bones. But when I died I too departed, simply and easily, unshackled from the old carcass just as smoothly as slipping and sliding down a greased chute. You drift out, much as air leaves a slow leak in a tire. And before you know it, there you are, ethereal and invisible, floating around as a packet of energy and essence. Oh you know who you are, and who you were but it doesn't seem to matter. You are disengaged from the anchor and free. And it dawns on you that it was only a temporary thing, this occupation of the cumbersome, burdensome, corporal being.

I noticed one important fact right away. I was lighter than air and in no time was ascending up above the trees, past the tallest canyons of buildings, into clouds that now seemed abrasive and richly textured. But it was a simple matter for me to sway and bend with the tides of turbulent winds, all the while steadily penetrating upward until I broke through the clouds into the warm and refreshingly clear upper atmosphere and beyond. Much as a balloon will float to an altitude which balances its buoyancy forces, so too I found my level in a region far from earth. And there to my surprise I found kindred souls, all of us units of energy and consciousness, identifiable by these characteristics much as before, when we knew each other by height, weight, skin color and voice. Depending on your energy density, you might settle in one region or another, nearer to or further from the earth and hence closer to or farther from the sun.

We live here for an indefinite period as far as I can tell. We'll stay until our energy levels are depleted, I'm told. And then? Well no one seems to know what comes next except there is a rumor that after the fun and relaxation of this new life, we are to be assigned another mission on earth (by God who is in charge) though no one can remember any previous transfers. It seems here we energy packets have no memories.

Chapter 2

In God We Trust

I. George was just an ordinary carbon atom, not too heavy, not too tall. His weight was exactly 12.01, the same as most of his fellow carbons. His spin orbitals were properly arranged, with two electrons in his inner K shell and four unpaired electrons in the L shell. His nucleus contained six neutrons and six protons as required, all nicely packed. Sure he knew some carbon atoms who were a little heavier, but they only constituted about one percent of all the carbons. George found contentment in knowing that he and his kind were very constant.

And they were everywhere, these carbon atoms, among the other hundred or more kinds of atoms in the world. Unlike the noble atoms like helium, neon and argon who disdained to join with the other atoms, carbons could be either alone and free and unattached or combined and married to other atoms to form family units. Alone, or joined to other carbon atoms, they could form the very durable and organized bonds of diamond or the less ordered, softer structure of graphite. Everyone said that the married carbon atoms were the fulfilled ones, for in marriage they transcended themselves and became part of an almost infinite variety of family units, each distinctive in size and weight and activity. Some, like the carbon-oxygen family were light and adventurous and floated beyond their substrate. Others when combined with metal atoms and other units became heavy and large and conservative and hardly capable of moving from one neighborhood to another.

It was a simple life which George (the ordinary carbon atom) led; mostly he was concerned with maintaining a stable, resting state for his electrons, trying to control his energy and avoiding those unseen forces which could destroy him. But this wasn't easy, for in the world there were mysterious forces at work which could disrupt his life. In ways which he and his fellow carbon atoms did not comprehend, and at unpredictable times there would be unleashed from the heavens, storms of energy, sometimes as electrical flashes, and sometimes as great vibrations. Very destructive and dangerous were the high speed helium atoms, which could rip you apart. So could high speed electrons. And there was gamma radiation, the electromagnetic waves. In waves and quanta these pulses of energy would come, blanketing the world as if some holocaust was about to descend. But not everyone was affected. (Certainly the imperious, noble helium, argon and neon would be immune.) While most of the atoms shuddered during these storms, the unlucky ones were mesmerized and then activated. Their electrons jumped, their nuclei quivered as if in transfiguration, and in a frenzy they mated and formed family units. Now separated from their past, these new compounds no longer resembled their old cohorts. Sometimes the family units, in some preordained ritual, would join forces in a communal existence, sharing their new bonds.

George was a religious atom, as were most of the atoms he knew. He believed in an organized universe with his God in control. He accepted his life as an atom philosophically and was willing to be mated when his time came. He had blissful confidence that God was good, and that there was a hereafter. If God chose George to be mated, he would go willingly. He knew that ultimately God would return him to his single state. So George was a believer and found the inner strength to endure. Those terrible storms which arose from time to time were acts of God; God has a purpose.

On this warm and sunny summer day, at this time in history, George a carbon atom in amorphous association with his colleagues in a charcoal briquet, was thrust upon a metal grid, doused with a volatile liquid, exposed to a lit match and engulfed in searing flames.

"My God, why have you chosen me for your torture?" cried George. His electrons were excited, the stress of heat and temperature produced an instability that suggested the end of the world. And when it seemed that he would not survive, two oxygen atoms, also excited and vibrating sympathetically were suddenly there, with their electrons bound to his. And they were mated to produce carbon dioxide.

To be a carbon dioxide molecule is to be a colorless gas, representing a small elite group on earth. For George it meant a loss of identity, a subordination of his personality for the good of his family, and a sharing of his electrons which were so precious to him. But despite these compromises, and even allowing for the loss of his carbon cohorts, there was a positive side to his marriage; he was no longer a one-dimensional character, no longer immobilized. He could soar with the wind, dive into liquids and dissolve, diffuse through membranes and do things he never dreamed were possible. "God has been good to me; I am seeing and experiencing miracles," he thought. "The God that brought the fire which caused me to suffer so much must have been testing me. He found me worthy, for have I not led a devout life. Now he has brought beautiful oxygens to my side. Surely God is good."

But the freedom which George and his oxygens felt, the euphoric flights were to be short-lived. Unnoticed near the flames were immense mountains which alternately expanded and contracted, inhaling and exhaling huge quantities of air in the process and generating terrible wind storms. It was during one of these cycles that George was sucked into the cavernous interior of one of the mountains, pressed against the moist, sticky walls by the vacuum and forced through the membrane which was the outer layer of the walls and dumped into one of the cells.

Then the attack by exotic molecules began. First it was a pyruvic acid molecule, which surrounded George and his oxygens. Aided and abetted by catalysts which drained George of his resistive energy, the pyruvics easily weakened the bonds between George and his oxygens and dissolved the marriage. In the ensuing confusion there were some rapid rearrangements and when the struggle was over, George and his oxygens were tied to a pyruvic acid molecule. It was just the beginning of the nightmare for George, who now was being whirled rapidly and unstoppably in the cell. In this roller-coaster ride in the cell he mated temporarily with hydrogen and water, lost electrons and got them back, and was subjected to deforming physical stresses—until, dizzy and exhausted, George regained his senses to find himself part of an almost infinite sea of carbons, oxygens, nitrogens, phosphoruses and hydrogens. He was now but one miniscule part of a DNA molecule, one carbon atom bound to thousands of others in chains and helices, in a chemical prison. "Being part of DNA is to be the controller of the life process," George was told. "We make the food and building blocks and supply the genes who enable our cell to survive and reproduce. Every atom is critical."

So he was welcomed to the team, with a warning, "No independence is allowed here; all must work for the common good. Get out of line or neglect the instructions being passed on by the messengers, and the whole process is upset. No mutants are tolerated in this cell, so there can be no laxity. We are all comrades."

II. To be a virus is to be someone who cannot reproduce with your own kind. To be a virus is to be a parasite, living in host cells which supply your food for life and the means for reproduction. To be a virus is to be about one-twentieth of the size of the smallest organism capable of independent reproduction. It's not an easy life. You must live by your wits, but a virus is immortal as long as one of its species survives. Let one enter a host cell and identical viruses will be produced. Though new, they are the same as the old.

Mary accepted her life as a smallpox virus. She was larger than most and heavier. With a brick-like shape which gave her strength and a hexagonal protein head containing DNA (which was the reason for her intelligence), Mary could compete easily for the host cells against the other viruses who had poor quality RNA in their heads and weaker shapes.

She was born in a lung cell and quickly understood the peculiar existence of her kind—not being able to eat or engage in sexual activities in the usual way. To be with your fellow smallpox viruses was to look at your own image in a mirror. Why viruses were destined for this kind of life Mary attributed to the design of God.

"The God that invented the virus also created bacteria and the cells, so the virus could survive," she often said. "The God which causes the flames and heat which kill viruses also gives them special shapes for survival. And when God brings a plague of antibodies to destroy us in the blood streams, there must be a reason. He intends us no permanent harm, for he also causes the virus to become immune to these same antibodies, guaranteeing our survival. Though there will be times when living conditions become intolerable, God will always provide the means for survival; viruses are the chosen ones." Mary believed in God, in His wisdom and omnipotence.

Mary the smallpox virus, born in a lung cell with hundreds of her sisters, in response to some primordial pressure, broke out of the cell of her birth and settled onto the exposed surface of the living lung. There she rested but briefly, for suddenly the ground wrenched, a distant rumble became audible and the wind velocity increased. Hugging the surface with her powerful legs, Mary cringed in fear of this irrational event, a storm which threatened her life. In a fraction of a second a perfectly calm day produced a cataclysmic burst of wind which swept her out of her home and into the air. She had been expelled from the land of her birth by forces governed by her God, for reasons unknown to her.

Sailing through the air, seemingly weightless, Mary had time to observe this new world. In some frightening way she was exhilarated by the danger and freedom, neither cancelling the other exactly. "Has God a special mission for me?" she wondered as she floated by a charcoal grill which was aflame. The heat was intense but she was beyond its reach. "I don't have much time to find a home. Where will I land?"

Mountain ranges loomed before her, positioned uniformly around the flames. Mary marvelled at the symmetry of the landscape, thoroughly enchanted with the new vistas and unaware that she was rapidly approaching one of the mountains. She didn't notice the periodic updraft which was drawing her toward the mountain top. The suction was getting stronger, the turbulent wind velocities were accelerating, her speed was increasing and she was now being buffeted badly. The joy of floating in this new world rapidly gave way to despair and an ineffective attempt to stabilize her flight. Sensing the hopelessness of her struggle, aware of the God-like dimensions of the forces at work, she succumbed to their will.

Mary did not crash into the mountain, but was swept instead into one of its cavities, impelled by a vacuum which also drew air, other viruses and bacteria. She crashed onto a lung surface and instinctively burrowed into its interstices. "I'll be safe from the wind here, but my strength won't hold up much longer without a host cell," she thought. "I seem to have done this before; all this seems so familiar." It was as if she were programmed by some grand designer.

Looking only for something familiar and comfortable she finally contacted a cell—a lung cell—and was surprised when the physical contact kindled a sexual stimulation previously unknown to her. Through her pores Mary exuded an enzyme which weakened the host cell's membrane and rendered it more permeable. With her legs firmly attached to the cell she squatted, contracting the external sheath of her body and allowing her inner tube to penetrate the cell membrane. Now straining mightily, with a killing effort, Mary drained the DNA genetic material from her head, through her body tube and into the host cell. The process took only one minute but now Mary understood that this was her reason for existing. Through her the smallpox virus would continue to live: God had chosen her for the most important function of the universe. She also knew that by her act she would die, for stripped of her DNA she was nothing. But death meant others would be born soon in her image. From Mary would come hundreds of smallpox viruses and she would be reborn. Hallelujah! She was immortal!

Old Mary died, but her DNA seeds were firmly implanted inside the host cell. Within minutes, the carbon atoms, the oxygens, nitrogens, phosphoruses and hydrogens of her DNA essence spread into the genes of the host cell. In less than one hour they had found their counterparts and had taken over the operation of the cell. Where formerly the DNA of the host cell had peacefully manufactured replacement parts, now they were overcome and the process was shut off. Instead of a pastoral existence, they were bullied into producing replicas of the smallpox virus, under exact instructions from Mary's messengers. First the DNA was to be assembled and condensed into a head. Next the legs and body were to be made and finally everything had to be covered with a protein coat. It took a few hours to complete the operation and now hundreds of new Marys were contained within the spent host cell. Old Mary was dead, young Mary lived.

"A carbon atom is passive by nature," said George to a fellow atom as they worked on the DNA assembly line. "We're usually unreactive unless highly stimulated. I accepted my fate when God converted me to carbon dioxide, and I can see a purpose in His drafting me into the DNA of this cell. The work is dull here but at least I feel part of a team. And we seem to be doing useful work. But when those dreadful smallpox atoms come in and force us to do their work, that's going too far. I will not build Mary viruses; these smallpox viruses are evil monsters who live parasitic lives, draining the life out of docile cells in their effort to proliferate. These fascists are also trying to force me to join one of their DNA molecules and become part of them. I'll not do it!"

But George didn't have much choice in the matter. He was forced to do the bidding of the smallpox messengers, assembling their DNA, until about halfway through one production run when the orders came for George to join the DNA which was being assembled as the head of a Mary virus. There is no resistance to such instructions since a virus enzyme is always present to break the bonds of recalcitrant atoms. So George the carbon atom was integrated into a smallpox virus.

"God is surely testing me in this new role he has chosen for me," said George, unhappily. "These are Godless creatures, and for me to aid in their destructive activities is offensive. I am a prisoner for reasons which God only knows."

Young Mary was beginning to stir, sensing that she was now complete as a smallpox virus.

"Thank you, God, for continuing the miracle of creation which proves that you are happy with us," she said. "I hope I may be worthy of your trust and can carry out your wishes. I pledge my DNA to your service."

George and Mary, Mary and George, were inseparable. George in slave labor, working against his will in the smallpox DNA helix, did his job as carbon atoms must. No carbon atom is unstable; carbon atoms do not break their bonds easily. He prayed that God would rescue him and restore his freedom. Young Mary, full of early bloom, energetic and fearless, probed at the host cell's surrounding membrane in an effort to escape. She found a weakness in the membrane of this dying cell and easily plunged through, ready for adventure.

"God give me the strength and courage to persevere," she said as she emerged from the cell.

III. Mark had enjoyed sitting around the charcoal grill with his fellow students, eating the hamburgers and chicken they cooked. All of them were new to the university so it was fun to swap horror stories about registration difficulties and new professors. They represented the U.N. in microcosm, having come from so many different countries. One of the animated discussions they had that day was about religion, and whose was best. The Buddhists, Muslims, Hindus, Christians and Jews made their representations and when it was over, they agreed to disagree, each strongly determined that his religion was best (and contained the only truth about God).

Ever since that picnic a week ago, Mark felt a bit feverish, and now he noticed that chills, shaky spells and restlessness were added to his symptoms. He awoke one day with a severe backache, vomited and found he had a temperature of 105 degrees. There were faint, irregular blotches on his skin. His doctor told him the bad news: he had contracted smallpox; apparently his lungs were the primary infection site.

"What rotten luck," Mark said to the doctor, knowing he would now have to miss some critical classes at the university. "How the hell did I get it?"

"Probably through one of the fellows from India or Africa or South America who were with you the day of your picnic."

"God is punishing me for not defending him more forcefully," Mark said sardonically.

The smallpox infection proved to be more virulent than they suspected; Mark had hemorrhagic smallpox which specifically affects the lungs and is the most dangerous form of the disease. In addition to the general symptoms and the skin lesions, and the damage to the liver and spleen, there is bleeding in the lungs with pneumonia arising as a secondary infection. Mark had never been in good health; as a student away from his parents he had further weakened himself by eating poorly. Thus this attack of smallpox became a very serious matter. Despite the best of medical care, despite inoculations to counteract the smallpox virus, Mark gradually slipped into a coma, the viruses now too entrenched to be overcome by Mark's antibodies. He died two weeks after the initial infection.

"Why has God punished us?" asked his parents. "Mark was so young, so full of promise. His whole life was before him; there was so much he wanted to do with his life. What kind of God is this?"

"Isn't it ironic," said the mourners, "how it's always the good people whom God chooses to die early."

"Our duty is not to question God's will," replied the others. "He has a purpose, even if it's not obvious to us."

(No one asked whose God had killed Mark—whether it was the God of Buddha, or Jesus or Abraham. Or was it Mary's God or George's? So they laid Mark into the ground, hoping for a sign that this death was in God's name and would be for the betterment of mankind.)

IV. Oh, how merry they were. A perfect climate for Mary viruses, they moved into one cell after another of Mark's lungs, organizing this cell and that one, generating more and more smallpox viruses at an accelerating rate. (George, on the DNA assembly line, was forced to work at a maddening pace, hardly daring to rest or think; there was only time to follow the orders of the messengers.) Everyone was so busy and full of robust health during those two weeks they didn't notice that the cells they invaded possessed increasingly sluggish DNA. Soon George and the others were having a difficult time converting the host cell's DNA for the manufacture of Mary viruses.

And then the alarm went out, "The new cells are not operable! The new cells can no longer be organized to produce smallpox."

And then the panic developed, "We'll starve unless we find more cells!"

They foraged in the liver and spleen, travelled the entire arterial and venus routes and even tried the lymphatics. It wasn't easy, moving through blood and lymph fluids, for then they were vulnerable to attacks by the antibodies. But their ranks were swollen by the urgency of their predicament and Mark's antibodies were unable to eliminate all the Mary viruses.

Two weeks after Mark was invaded by Mary he died rendering all of Mary's host cells useless. The bacterial flora from Mark's intestines now migrated to the lymphatics, blood capillaries and veins and finally into body tissue including the respiratory system. The aerobic bacteria used up the available oxygen, allowing the anaerobic bacteria coming mostly from the intestines to begin their proliferation. New forces were now at work; strange enzymes and chemicals appeared which were obnoxious to Mary. The new bacteria which appeared were immune to Mary's enzymes. The world was collapsing; they were on the verge of disaster. Chemical bonds which were unbreakable before, now crumbled before the new enzymes. With no host cells and a toxic environment, the smallpox viruses began to die in hordes. Some even became cannibalistic and attacked each other in their death frenzy.

"The God who was so good has turned on us," said Mary. "This ugliness He has given us must be punishment for some offense we have committed against Him. Surely there must be a reason for this cruelty."

The Mary viruses died seeking some sign from God.

"Thank God the smallpox viruses have been destroyed," said George. "I had my doubts about Him, but I guess we atoms can't comprehend the infinity of God's deeds."

The new enzymes broke George's DNA bonds and liberated him. He eventually mated with four hydrogens to become an odorless, colorless, gaseous methane molecule and floated away from the crumbling smallpox milieu, up through the earth of Mark's grave into the free air.

"Once again a gas? Isn't this a bit redundant?" George thought. The sensuality of his new marriage to the hydrogens was dampened by the memory of his previous experience. George was thankful for his release from the Mary virus but remained leery.

"I'll do God's bidding, but I hope He chooses someone else."

George's methane family, driven by the winds, drifted about the earth, settling occasionally in a coal mine or a pool of stagnant water or some sewage. (Within the time frame of the universe it was a relatively short time.) And finally, at a time unmarked, in a place unknown, lightning flashed at George. The searing heat tore at George's methane bonds and in the presence of a few oxygens, caused a chemical reaction to form free carbon and two water molecules. The odyssey was ended, George was again a free carbon atom.

"Thank God."

V. Alice loved to play with her Milky Way, her pinwheel-shaped galaxy with its five spiral arms, a flattened disc of two billion stars, gases and cosmic dust. She delighted in displacing the constellation Sagittarius from its center position, a movement which produced resonances within the Milky Way and upset the fine balance of magnetic and electrical forces. This in turn would alter the distance of Sagittarius from the earth's sun, causing sun spots which affected tiny earth so interestingly.

God has been good to Alice.

Chapter 3

Longevity: Theories and Speculation

How old are you?

How do you know?

Who is older, you or I?

How old are your lungs? Your heart? Eyes? Skin? Hair?

There's a difference, you know.

And a variability to lifespan. Man versus woman, between animals, trees, corporations and civilizations.

Can you hear time flying? Listen to the silence. Do you hear the clock ticking away, tolling the beginning, the middle, and the end? Hey, rabbit in my garden, do you know that you will die in a year or two? That your lifespan is clearly circumscribed? Do you ever talk of these things with your brothers and sisters as you munch on the sweet green leaves which taste so good?

Everyone gets nervous when we talk of aging. Don't tell me I'm going to die. I won't hear of it. But something is going on. Changes are occurring so at eighty your heart can pump blood only at about half of what it could do at age sixty.[1] Body temperature is down.But the Bristlecone Pine tree can live to 4,000 years; some even to 4,600 years. A fly may live a day; a flea, 30 days; a white rat, 4 years; dogs and cats, 20 years; chimpanzees and horses, 40 years; hippopotamuses, 50 years; Indian elephants, 80 years; fresh water mussels and some fish, 100 years; large tortoises, 150 years.

---

1. Langone, J., Long life, Little, Brown & Company, Boston, 1978

Cro-Magnum man believed a cave painting held the soul of the subject. Aztec souls went to the sun. Borneo natives inferred seven souls in every body; that these fly from us at death through the big toe in the shape of a butterfly. Buddhists had an Eightfold Path of Righteous Living: death and life and death, again and again, until we wend our way through a long chain of rebirths to Nirvana. The Muslims prescribe a Heaven of Sensual Delight. The Greeks poured wine on the fresh graves during burial and sacrificed animals to feed the resident souls—and envisioned the Elysian Fields, located by Homer on the western border of earth. The alchemists considered that the sun ruled the heart, the moon the brain, Jupiter the liver, Saturn the spleen, Mercury the lungs, Mars the bile, Venus the kidneys.

We yearn for immortality. Don't you? At least can't we have a long life in good health, with our senses and strengths unimpaired, with sufficient money to enjoy the good life? And if we suffer some losses, why can't we rejuvenate our being, especially our sexual powers and appearance? Throughout history we have sought the magical cure, the extract from our vital organs which when ingested or injected, provides the restorative healing capability. Our modern research, though disguised and bearing the cachet of scientific respectability nevertheless continues in the vein of our ancient predecessors, exploring the effects of nutrients or hormones on lifespan. Injecting spleen cells from young mice into old mice can extend longevity by one-third in some cases. Something called antabotone extracted from the squirrel's brain lowers the body temperature of rats about five degrees, apparently slowing the metabolic processes and extending their tenure. Diminishing the fruit fly temperature from 25°C to 19°C seems to double its lifespan. Rotifers react similarly. For people, lowering body temperature by two degrees decreases our basal metabolic rate by 8 percent. Conversely, wound healing is improved by raising the temperature; higher temperatures also accelerate the destruction of invading bacteria and viruses by cells called phagocytes. A chemical called monoamine oxidase in the brain seems to be related to depression and schizophrenia. Treat these disorders by suppressing the levels of monoamine oxidase is the thinking today. Or is it the immune system which is the cause of our demise: old people die of infection and the complications derived therefrom, say the researchers today who seek ways of bolstering the immune surveillance system. Remove the thymus and you decrease the concentration of the hormone thymosin and retard the immune system. A lack of suppressor cells is thought to allow an uncontrolled antibody production. This may or may not be advantageous for us; on the one hand we need the antibodies to fight disease, yet on the other hand these excesses may lead to deranged antibodies which attack our own cells, a masochist's dream, resulting in the autoimmune diseases of old age such as lupus erythematosis.

None of the foregoing ideas and observations provide the answer to the recondite question as to *the* cause of aging, but considering them in toto, perhaps we can surround the unknown, this black hole of knowledge—where everything we do, all questions asked, get devoured; where no solutions emerge. One of my favorite theories of aging, the free radical theory[1], says that there are certain parts of molecules—free radicals—which are ephemeral, transitory, very unstable, highly reactive and therefore eminently disruptive to the chemistry of life in our bodies. They enter into our vital oxygen reactions, form side products which are unneeded or noxious, weaken cell membranes, disturb the delicate DNA machinery and in general produce weakened cells and organs. Radiation exposure as well as oxygen and ozone are thought to be free radical generators. The animal or person exposed to radiation suffers the apparent effects of an accelerated aging process: thickened artery linings; wrinkled skin; and accumulation of so-called old age pigments such as lipofuscin and amyloid. A small animal can be killed by high

---

1. Hershey, D., Lifespan and factors affecting it, Thomas, Springfield, Ill., 1974

concentrations of ozone; the astronauts in the early days of the U.S. space program suffered eye problems when exposed to a pure oxygen environment. We are asked to eat more unsaturated (soft) fats in order to prevent heart disease yet we now know that free radicals are more easily generated by the unsaturated fats, as opposed to the hard, saturated variety. Hence the dilemma for us: if all this is true, if by the very nature of living, in the course of normal existence, we generate these harmful free radicals, then first of all why do we humans tend to live so long and secondly can't we do something to neutralize the free radicals. The explanations offered are glib, unproved and provocative. We live our lives, we die our deaths in a controlled manner; the rate of living is moderated by naturally occurring free radical scavengers residing within the cells of our bodies and concomitantly we ingest foods containing these same free radical neutralizers (also called antioxidants). Vitamin E is one of them, so are vitamins A and C as well as a class of chemicals called mercaptans and others with abstruse nomenclature—BHT, 2-MEA, Santoquin. In the diets of rats, these free radical scavengers (antioxidants) enabled the experimental group to outlive the control. If true, if free radicals are the bane of our existence, if we can slow their formation, if we can demonstrate that by diminishing the presence of copper (the catalytic agent of the free radical reaction) we live longer, then will you become a believer or shall we dig further into the molecular realm and ask what is the ultimate agent causing free radicals to appear.

Collagen is a protein material which forms the structural component of our bodies and also the surfaces through which diffuse the enzymes, vital oxygen and other sources of life. In its youthful condition, collagen is soluble in some fluids and appears to be fibrous or stringy under the microscope. With time, young collagen becomes old collagen and insoluble, cross-linked and stiffer than before. And so, you and I as we age, get stiffer, more prone to pull an Achilles' tendon if not "warmed up" or stretched sufficiently before exercising.

We get less oxygen through our lung surfaces when old for these membranes are mostly collagen; it also becomes more difficult to take a deep breath. Literally painful to do. And so we slow down, stiffen, confined as we are in an ever tightening straightjacket of old collagen, unable to inhale our optimum amounts of oxygen, our vitality diminished, ripe for the other debilitating scourges of old age. Remember the professional football player a few years ago, the quarterback who at age 39 (advanced for this sport), with a history of lackadaisical attention to physical conditioning programs, walked onto the practice field for the first time in a new season, threw one football and tore his Achilles' tendon? Out for the season and at the end of his career, our star was a victim of old, cross-linked collagen. If you believe this collagen or cross-linking theory of aging, then you may ask, "Where do we find the cure?" What we seek is the magic bullet, a bacterium or virus inclined to devour old collagen. We know they exist for they work quite effectively in soils when our bodies are finally laid to rest there. But there must be a certain specificity for it is the cross-linked, insoluble, inflexible collagen we wish to remove, thereby providing the space for our bodies to lay down a nascent mesh of young, soluble, flexible fibrils. In the meantime, until the panacea is found, we must be content to contemplate the tantalizing, incomplete research results which seem to indicate that a free radical neutralizer such as vitamin C is effective in ameliorating the effects of cross-linking of collagen. Indeed there is some evidence suggesting that old people lose their teeth not so much through tooth decay, but because of shrinking gums (composed of collagen) and the subsequent exposure of tooth roots which yield ultimately a loosening and detachment of the teeth from their bases. Vitamin C is a factor in preventing the cross-linking and shrinking of the gums and associated tooth loss.

The wear and tear (rate of living) theory of aging[1] expresses the conviction that just as the machine wears out, the living system does also. (Survival curves for

---
1. Hershey, D., op. cited

automobiles, cockroaches and people are similarly shaped.) Gasoline fuels the engine, food energizes the body. There is a certain prescribed duration of light which can emanate from a lightbulb in its lifetime (the rating is prominently displayed on the container); shouldn't we expect the same limitation for an animate system in terms of its complement of energy, enzymes or other vital matters and can't we project a longevity in proportion to the levels of these resources at birth and the rate at which they are consumed? Finally, ultimately, couldn't we expect senile death to approach when the energy or enzymes are depleted or reach a critically low level of concentration? This then is the essence of the wear and tear or rate of living theory of aging. Aided and abetted by fascinating empirical observations, the apostles of this cause are firm in their convictions. For example, in experiments done thirty and forty years ago and verified readily since then, rats were underfed—healthy diets but lacking in the caloric content of the control group—and when the lifespans were totaled, the underfed rats lived longer. The feeding regimen could be altered, one day of fasting in a three-day cycle didn't change the results. In different experiments, the heartbeats were summed for rats and elephants. The rats, living two or three years, with heart rates of about 500 beats per minute generated approximately one billion beats in an average lifetime; the elephants, 25 beats per minute, living to about 80 years of age also averaged approximately one billion heartbeats. And then there are the cell doubling experiments: cells taken from the youngest human living, fetal tissue could double around fifty times before the cell population senesced and died. Obtaining cells from a mature person and performing the same doubling experiments yielded only twenty doublings before the population dissipated itself. Indeed the experiment could be refined by removing those youngest cells from their milieu after ten doublings, freezing them in a liquid nitrogen bath, distributing them around the world to other laboratories, waiting six years, thawing the cells and resuming the protocol. Those youngest cells, with an initial potential of fifty doublings, having already doubled ten times, after six years resumed their splittings for about forty more times. Curiously, cells from subjects with cystic fibrosis exhibited normal population doublings in early passages. However, after about thirteen doublings these cells began to double more slowly than the control group and ceased doubling after nineteen compared to twenty-seven for the control. It may be that these cells of cystic fibrosis patients were demonstrating some sort of premature aging syndrome.[1] Dramatic stuff—cell doublings, heartbeats, underfeeding—and perfect support for the wear and tear (rate of living) enthusiasts.

These then are the essential theories of aging. Aided and abetted by tangential but no less important new developments related to the control processes within the brain, we are beginning to understand the grand ensemble. The evolving immune system function with age is an example of the control thought to be exercised by the brain.[2] The brain is the origin, from which is derived an understanding of the hypothalamus (governs the pituitary gland, hunger, satiety, body temperature, water balance, blood pressure, heart rate), the pituitary (influences metabolism, growth, reproduction), the thyroid (affects metabolism, oxygen consumption) and the thymus (generates the essence of the immune system). All of these functions are dependent upon neurotransmitters such as dopamine, serotonin and acetylcholine, affecting the transmission of nerve signals. The level of dopamine in the brain is known to diminish with age, a fact uncovered when attention was riveted on it as a treatment for Parkinson's disease. Found in such foods as wheat germ and velvet beans, L-dopa becomes dopamine in our bodies. It affects the aging process or the symptoms of aging in ways not yet

---

1. Shapiro, B.L., L.R.H. Lam, L.H. Fast, Premature senescence in cultured skin fibroblasts from subjects with cystic fibrosis, Science Vol. 203, 1979, 1251-3
2. Rosenfeld, A., Prolongevity, Knopf, New York, 1976

clearly specified except that we know its absence affects hypothalamus function. The thyroid in the neck area has been the focus of attention for half a century or more, in the study of conditions associated with the underproduction or overproduction of the hormone thyroxine which is secreted by the thyroid. Too little thyroxine diffusing into the cells causes the basal metabolic rate to be insufficient for proper energy metabolism. The patient seems listless and deenervated. Too high a level of thyroxine revs up the cells, developing a hyperactive and hence inefficient operation. Hypothyroidic persons tend to have too many wrinkles, grey hair, low resistance to disease, retarded growth and weakened muscle and cardiovascular function. Hyperthyroid cases exhibit nervousness, decreased growth and shortened lifespan. Old persons in good health generally show no abnormally high or low levels of thyroxine in their blood. This was a seeming paradox until it was established that the problem was not concentrations in the blood but the inability of the thyroxine to penetrate the enveloping cell membrane. Even with normal thyroid function and acceptable levels of thyroxine in the blood, this energizing hormone thyroxine is apparently unable to diffuse into the cells in proper amounts. The result is a rundown system, not operating at its proper level, contributing to the common observation that old folks' basal metabolic rates drop steadily with age, their vitality is diminished monotonically and they become more prone to be victims of killing stresses such as disease, physical injury, psychological traumas and other vectors younger persons are able to shrug off. There is some evidence that this increasing inability to get thyroxine into the cells is a programmed event, orchestrated by the pituitary. Something is excreted from the pituitary in our mature and later phases of life which seems to block the movement of thyroxine. Ominously called the "death hormone", its presence (though not its identification) has been indicated indirectly. By excising the pituitary of some old rats and then adding thyroxine to the bloodstream, the debilitating effects of a thyroxine lack are reversed; the rats become seemingly rejuvenated. Nothing is really proved here yet, only a clue and a tentative one to be sure. Find a way to neutralize this so-called death hormone, find a way to facilely get thyroxine into the cells of old folks and you will create a revolution. Think of it: elderly people who are strong and vital. Remember the discussion of underfeeding and its effect on lifespan? Suppose underfeeding maintains the pituitary in a youthful condition, delaying the time when, if you believe those who say these events are programmed, the death hormone is released. Do we live longer on a restricted diet because this affects the pituitary in a way which delays or reduces the secretion of the death hormone, which then allows the cells to accept more thyroxine, improving cell energy metabolism?

The acolytes of the immune theory of aging focus on the thymus. Here is located the essence of the immune system, they believe. The thymus receives cells from the bone marrow (B or bone marrow derived cells) and through action with the hormone thymosin secreted by the thymus, causes the development of T or thymus derived cells. The T cells stimulate the continued production of B cells by some sort of feedback mechanism as yet not understood and enter the blood and lymphoid tissue to become killer cells (lymphocytes) capable of attacking cancer cells, viruses and bacteria. The B cells from the bone marrow differentiate to lymphocytes and also enter lymphoid tissue. They secrete antibody molecules which provide immunity against disease-causing germs. The thymus atrophies at an early age, shortly after puberty in humans. B cell function declines shortly thereafter. T cells seem to change most with age, exhibiting early difficulty in dividing. Their loss in function is believed to affect B cell antibody secretion, leading to an increased presence of deranged antibodies called autoantibodies which attack our own body's tissue. Old people have elevated levels of autoantibodies, and suffer from what are believed to be autoimmune diseases: rheumatoid arthritis and maturity onset diabetes.

Harrison[1] examined food restriction and parabiosis (the joining of the blood circulatory systems of two animals) as they affect immunological aging in mice. He found that food restriction appeared to slow the loss in immune function with age. Parabiosis did not rejuvenate the old, and at the same time suggested something within the old organism had a negative effect upon the younger mice.

Tolmosoff, et. al.[2] address themselves to the free radical theory of aging and suggest the superoxide free radical as the debilitating influence. Attention has focused recently on superoxide dismutase (SOD), the neutralizer of the superoxide free radical. SOD may remove the superoxide free radical. Its presence has been established in the liver, brain, the heart of rodents and primates including man. We humans seem to have the highest levels of SOD. Longer-lived species may have a higher degree of SOD protection against the by-products of the oxygen metabolism which yields superoxide free radicals. Is it possible that soon the new wonder drug will be SOD, to be taken by pill as easily as we ingest vitamins today? Tolmosoff, et. al. also suggest a maximum lifespan potential for us of about 110 years. They report maximum lifespan energy expenditures of 200 to 300 kilocalories per gram of body weight for many mammals; primates in general generate two times this amount and man the exception about three times as much.

Rodents dietarily restricted since weaning show strikingly extended lifespans, delayed onsets of the expected diseases of old age, younger performing immune systems in old age than the corresponding control group.[3] We know that the thymus is involved in the workings of the immune system. The thymus weight generally peaks

---

1. Harrison, D.C., Treatments that retard or reverse immunological losses with age, 32nd Gerontological Society Annual Scientific Meeting, Dallas, 1979
2. Tolmosoff, J.M., T. Ono, R.G. Cutler, Superoxide dismutase: correlation with lifespan and specific metabolic rate of primate species, personal communication.
3. Weindruck, R.H., S.C. Suffin, Dietary restriction and thymic history, submitted to the J. Gerontology, 1979

at puberty; long-lived mice attain their peak thymus weights later in life than do the shorter-lived strains. The weight loss is believed to be caused by a loss of cells, affecting the ability of the thymus to produce T cells. Removing the thymus of adult mice decreases longevity and seems to accelerate aging. Grafts of thymuses from young mice to old mice offer partial immunological rejuvenation as does treatment of old mice with a thymus extract, pentapeptide thymopoitin. The ability of thymus grafts to restore some immune responses of thymectocized (thymus removed) mice depends on the age of the donor: the younger the better. Dietarily restricted mice had thymuses which were younger structurally than the control group.[1] Apparently underfeeding is somehow able to maintain this organ, the thymus, in a youthful condition for longer timespans than otherwise and suggests future studies to establish whether this too is true for humans. Should we restrict the diet of our children —not aim for more rapid growth patterns—to produce a conservative, slower growing juvenile state?

Implicitly we are beginning to expand on the narrowly defined theories of aging. Should we use 24 physiological parameters as a measure of biological age[2] or segregate the theories along deterministic lines (longevity is a by-product of fitness, the failure of nature to eliminate imperfections, or a programmed degenerational process) and non-deterministic approaches (longevity is stochastic-based, depending on probability and random events which cause changes with time).[3] In other words, is aging programmed by our genes and the environment—or is it a natural evolutionary, chancy thing, whereby we expect life's chemistry to produce damage with time (it's bound to happen sooner or later).

1. Cheng, M.K., R.H. Weindruck, M.A. Verity, R.L. Walford, Effects of dietary restriction on mitochondrial respiration, Presented at the Gerontological Society 32nd annual meeting, Dallas, 1979.
2. Borkan, G.A., A.H. Norris, A new approach to biological assessment, presented at the Gerontological Society 32nd Annual Meeting, Dallas, 1979.
3. Mayer, P.J., The evolution of human longevity, presented at the Gerontological Society 32nd Annual Meeting, Dallas, 1979.

There were estimated to be 23 million people sixty-five years of age or older in the U.S. in 1979 (11% of the population)[1] whereas in 1900 the count was three million (4% of the population). If extrapolations are accurate, we could see 55 million in the year 2030. In the still older category, those over one-hundred years of age, Congressional figures show 13,000 today, as compared to 3,000 ten years ago. Health care expenditure in 1977 amounted to $413 billion for the over-sixty-five group (30 percent of the total cost for all of the U.S.). Per capita expenditures for the over-sixty-five group in 1977 was $1,745 compared to $661 for the 19 to 64 age category and $253 for those under 19 years of age. In light of these figures, the study of the aging process (the experiments aimed at elucidating the mechanisms of aging) becomes terribly important. The denouement, the payoff, is the amelioration and control of the debilitating aspects so that old people will be enabled to live their years in relative good health. Not only from scientific and humanistic points of view, but also from the economic and baldly pragmatic political aspects.

In one group over 80 years of age, where there was a good immune system, 35 percent were dead within two years whereas in that same group those with delayed or absent sensitivity to specific antibodies (a sluggish immune response system), 80 percent were gone within the same two year period. Eighty percent versus 35 percent. Senile dementia is severe in 5 percent of those over 65 years of age, mild to moderate in 10 percent. This means a loss of initiative, decreased judgement, difficulty in selecting words, loss of recent memory, difficulty in performing calculations, disorientation and personality deterioration. The search for reasons—for explanations—as to why senile dementia strikes some and not others is focused on the brain and the neurotransmitters of the brain, those chemicals which enhance the signal transmission capability. Acetylcholine is a neurotransmitter; it activates the synapses in the limbic system of

---

[1]. Dans, P.E., M.R. Kerr, Gerontology and geriatrics in medical education, The New England Journal of Medicine, Feb. 1, 1979, 228-232.

the brain, controlling such functions as memory. The enzyme which helps produce acetylchloline declines in concentration with age in the brain of persons suffering senile dementia in Alzheimer's disease. There is a 70 to 90 percent loss. Therefore, the syllogism goes: add neurotransmitters to the diet, find a way to maintain them at youthful levels in people and avoid senility. True or false. Perhaps the answer is a resounding maybe. So now we can think about adding neurotransmitters to the diet to assist brain and immune functions. And perhaps we can reduce caloric intake to slow the rate of living and again help our immune systems. Of course there are alternate hypothesis as to the biological mechanism affected by underfeeding.[1] If food restriction is not for you, will you jazz up your immune system with bee stings?[2] We'll have more on this later but consider the tantalizing fact that bee keepers are relatively free of rheumatoid arthritis and other immune diseases of old age.

The original questions still apply. How old are you? How do you know who is older, you or I? How old are your lungs, heart, etc.? We know our maximim work output declines at a greater rate compared to the individual organs of our body.[3] So the question becomes important: How old are you? What do you mean by the question? The whole may be older than the individual parts. In crank turning experiments, we suffer a greater loss as a whole than do the involved muscles. Similar conclusions for maximum breathing capacity vis-a-vis isolated lung function. Apparently the insults delivered to our organs has a cumulative effect, so that finally we see a reduction in our ability to tolerate sugars, a condition derived from a slightly lowered ability of the pancreas to respond to blood glucose concentrations. The senescent heart responds with increasing difficulty to catecholamine stimulation. There is a slower rate of relaxation in the old heart, yet there seems to be sufficient calcium ions present

---

1. D Hew News Release, Jan. 2, 1971, NIH, Irene Fred (301), 496-1752
2. Mraz, C., Personal communication, Oct. 17, 1978
3. Shock, N.W., Systems physiology and aging, Federation Proceedings, Vol. 38, No. 2, Feb. 1979, 161-2

after contraction to allow this. The unused portion of the lung volume increases with age in proportions beyond the range of change in collagen.

Let's not dwell on the losses. Instead we take cognizance of the free radical neutralizers (antioxidants) which when added to maternal mouse diets extend the lifespan of the offspring.[1] Thymosin has the ability to cause T cells to become active. In vitro (in laboratory glassware, outside of the living body) incubation of old lymphocytes with thymosin can restore their immune function.[2] Aging in rats is correlated with the fall in serum levels of vitamin C (an antioxidant) in the liver.[3] A decline in amounts of vitamin C in the spleen preceded the onset of autoimmune diseases. Females showed earlier declines and earlier autoimmune diseases. This information is exciting, for it suggests Promethean experiments we can do now, as soon as we can buy vitamin C tablets and set up a protocol. What if it is true, that restoring vitamin C levels in the blood to youthful levels will prevent autoimmune diseases and other decrepitudes. Would you volunteer for the program? Would you send your elderly parent?

Old people in the Caucasus mountains between the Black Sea and the Caspian Sea have been the object of much scientific and commercial interest (as yogurt salesmen). Another pocket of long-livers resides in the village of Vilcambia in the Equadorian Andes; a third settlement is found in the high valley of the Karakorum mountains of northernmost Kashmir at the extreme western end of the Himalayas. We on the outside are naturally curious about the common denominators distinctive to these geriatric ensembles, people who live

---

1. Harmon, D., D.E. Eddy, Free radical theory of aging. Effect of adding antioxidants to maternal mouse diets, presented at the Gerontological Society 32nd Annual Meeting, Dallas, 1979
2. Fujivara, P., A. Amman, D. Wara, M. Cowan, Aging and immuneologic function: In vitro lymphocyte response to thymosin, presented at the Gerontological Society 32nd annual meeting, Dallas, 1979
3. Leibovitz, B., B.V. Siegel, J.T. Morton, Tissue vitamin C levels as a function of ages in healthy and autoimmune mice, presented at the Gerontological Society 32nd annual meeting, Dallas, 1979

long lives in good health. We notice that the populations of these lands do hard physical labor. Their diets are low in calories. They continue to be active and respected, though aged—which seems so different from our modern, sophisticated societies. On closer scrutiny, however, some are not as old as they claim and isn't that a pity. It appears there was considerable falsification of birth dates and ages under the Czars and afterward, done for a number of reasons, including an attempt to avoid military service. During Stalin's time the Russians were quite anxious to please Stalin, a former resident of one of the pockets of long-livers. By association he could also claim to have an extended life potential. Despite studies of these peoples and other anthropological explorations, the theory—or theories—of long life have not advanced much beyond the ideas promulgated in 1889 by Brown-Sequard of the University of Paris, who believed our aging gonads were the key: testicular extracts should have a rejuvenation effect. By the 1920's Serge Vornoff of the College de France grafted sex glands from young non-human primates into aging humans. At the turn of the twentieth century Elie Metchnikoff, an associate of Louis Pasteur in Paris, theorized that aging was due to the effects of intestinal toxins. He advocated a diet rich in lactobacillis bulgaris (a bacterium in yogurt). A Russian, A.A. Bogomolets, invoked the collagen theory and found some sort of serum for revitalization of our connective tissue. Anna Aslan, in Roumania, for the past two decades has used Gerovital H3, a procaine material like the dentist's Novocain, for treatment whose aim is rejuvenation. It may be that Gerovital H3 is a weak inhibitor of monoamine oxidase and as such may affect the hypothalamus. Hans Selye at the University of Montreal claimed stress as the aging vector. Background radiation was the culprit according to physicist Leo Szilard when he was at the University of Chicago. Szilard suggested that radiation randomly impinged on our chromosomes, inducing the changes which produce a steadily weakened organism. Leslie Orgel in England authored an error or catastrophe theory, whereby the DNA protein synthesizing apparatus is damaged, yielding faulty templates for protein production. John Bjorksten in Wisconsin is the major proponent of the collagen or cross-linking theory of aging. C.M. McCay at Cornell, forty years ago prolonged the life of rats up to 25 percent by diet restriction in early life.

Max Rubner in 1908 totaled the number of calories consumed per gram of body weight during the lifespan of mammals and found the amount was approximately the same for the mouse (3.5 year lifespan) and the elephant (70 year lifespan). Cumulative heartbeats over these lifespans were amazingly similar, 1.1 billion and 1.0 billion respectively. Think about it, that mouse living so rapidly, for so short a duration and the dissimilar elephant—both have a rhythm of life in phase. Live faster, live less. Raymond Pearl at Johns Hopkins working with fruit flies during the early twentieth century found the environmental temperature to be a factor affecting lifespan. Raise the temperature, shorten the lifespan and vice versa. Women live about eight years longer than men, perhaps because they have basal metabolic rates about six percent below men. Bernard Strehler at the University of Southern California discovered that mice with depressed body temperatures live up to twice as long as others. A.V. Everett, an Australian, believed in a biological clock or pacemaker, as did Caleb Finch also at the University of Southern California. W.D. Denkla at the Harvard School of Medicine proposed a special hormone, a "death hormone", secreted from the pituitary which controls the thyroid and the thymus and hence the aging process. Leonard Hayflick's in vitro experiments demonstrated a limited clonal lifespan for human diploid cells.

We search for the means to maintain good health into old age, to eliminate early deaths, to reduce sharply deaths in the middle years and early old age where the encroachments of geriatric illnesses manifest themselves more obviously. The goal is to alter the survival curve from that of ancient Rome (20 percent dead by age 10; all gone by around 100 years of age) to the ideal case (none dead by age 10; few dead by age 80; rapid decrease in survivors from age 90 to 110). Survivor curves haven't changed very much since the days of ancient Rome, except that fewer children are dying in the early years. In 1900 the average life expectancy was about 46 and 48 years for men and women respectively; in 1976 the equivalent numbers were 68 and 76. However, though average life expectancy is increasing, our ultimate lifespan, the age attained by the last few survivors is and has been well over 100, stretching towards 105 to 110. It has not changed much in hundreds of years of history.

With age there is a decline in the concentration of the neurotransmitter, dopamine, thereby affecting the hypothalamus and indirectly the pituitary.[1] Let's dwell a bit on the neurotransmitters such as norepinephrine, dopamine and serotonin, particularly dopamine. Remember, the hypothalamus governs the pituitary, controls hunger, body temperature, water balance, blood pressure, heart rate. The pituitary is the nexus for metabolic growth and reproductive activity. Parkinson's disease is characterized by a dopamine deficiency, reversible in some patients simply by the administration of dopamine. In the hypothalamus, with age, there is a loss of dopamine in what is called the median eminence which is just above the pituitary. This region of the hypothalamus is believed to control the "releasing factors", hormones flowing to the pituitary. Feeding the precursor of dopamine, namely L-dopa, to mice gained a 10 percent life extension and many more than usual stayed healthy in later life (the ultimate goal of gerontological research). However, there are side effects accruing from the L-dopa treatment, including bouts of schizophrenia, a not always acceptable alternative to the original disease. L-dopa in rats reduced the incidence of mammary tumors and increased the release of gonadotrophin (influencing ovulation). Some breast cancers have been successfully treated with L-dopa.

---

1. Bylinsky, G., Science is on the trail of the fountain of youth, Fortune, July, 1976, 134-140

Let's focus on the thymus again. Recall that cells from the bone marrow migrate to the thymus and develop into T cell lymphocytes (killer cells) which attack cancer cells, viruses and bacteria. Some cells from the bone marrow travel to peripheral lymphoid tissue as B cell lymphocytes, producing antibody molecules that lock onto invading foreign objects. If something goes awry, we have not this efficient, well-balanced immune system but a deranged autoimmune response: lymphocytes attacking the host cells, a masochist's dream, and we destroy ourselves. Rheumatoid arthritis, anemia and kidney disease result. The battle against this withering process has a number of banner carriers, including legions of McCay followers who believe in underfeeding and others who transplant thymuses and bone marrow from young mice into old ones and achieve some sort of immune system rejuvenation. Some seek from the pituitary the aging or death hormone, released, they believe, after puberty. We know that the level of thyroxine, the hormone released by the thyroid, remains unchanged in old rats; rather it is the responsiveness of old cells to the thyroxine that troubles us, a decline of about 60 percent.

Apparently underfeeding slows the pituitary output including the death hormone, if it exists. Remove the pituitary in the old rat and achieve rejuvenation? Perhaps. Cut out the pituitary of some old rats, inject thyroxine and find a higher phagocyte level (cells which devour foreign material)? It's been done. And concomitantly, antibody production is restored as is fur growth.

The lexicon of researchers on the frontiers of knowledge in gerontology[1] includes Denham Harmon who demonstrated a life extension possibility by feeding mice 2-MEA (2-mercaptoethylamine), BHT (butylated hydroxytoluene), vitamin E and Santoquin (a quinoline derivative)—all of them free radical neutralizers or scavengers (antioxidants). We know that mothers fed antioxidants had long-lived offspring. Charles Barrows

---

1. Rosenfeld, A., Are we afraid of living longer, Saturday Review, May 27, 1978, 10-13

increased the longevity of rats by about 30 percent by halving the protein content in the feed of mature rats. Allan Goldstein of the University of Texas in Galveston injected thymosin into rats and boosted their immune function. Paul Chretien successfully used thymosin in lung cancer therapy in conjunction with chemotherapy. Others apply anti-aging concepts such as seeking temperature-lowering drugs, or experiment with L-dopa or collagen cross-linking inhibitors (vitamin C) or cell membrane stabilizers (selenium) or lipofuscin scavengers (antioxidants).

The octopus dies after spawning, as does the salmon. For the octopus, the corticosteroid hormones are released by the optic nerve. Remove the optic nerve and you can double the lifespan of the female octopus. Harman[1] claims a diet containing free radical scavengers (antioxidants) has increased the lifespan of mice, rats and fruit flies, inhibited some forms of cancer, allowed less deposition of the yellow old age pigment, amyloid, and increased the immune response. The proper diet can add 5 to 10 years of life, he claims. The damage inflicted by free radical reactions are: (1) cross-linking of collagen and elastin, the structural protein of the body; (2) breakdown of the membrane and cell material through which oxygen, enzymes and other vital substances diffuse; (3) accumulation of aging pigments by polymerization of lipids and proteins; (4) changes in mitochondria membranes by excess oxidation (peroxidation) and (5) thickening of the small blood vessel walls (fibrosis) by oxidation of the blood serum and the wall linings. A very damaging free radical reaction involves the superoxide free radical. Luckily the enzyme superoxide dismutase (SOD) has the capacity to remove the superoxide presence. By caloric restriction we can lower the level of free radical reactions. By minimizing copper levels in our body free radical reactions may be slowed (copper is part of the catalyst which helps generate the reactions). By eating less polyunsaturated fats we can accomplish the same results

---

1. Harman, D., Free radical theory of aging: nutritional implications, Age, Vol. 1, Oct., 1978, 145-152

(polyunsaturated fats produce free radical enhancing peroxides when metabolized). By adding to our diets free radical scavengers such as 2-MEA, α-tocopherol (vitamin E), BHT and Santoquin we can attenuate the free radical reactions. Thinner people should live longer—restricted diets for rats soon after weaning produced about a 40 percent increase in lifespan—with the onset of old age diseases delayed. Easily oxidized amino acids such as histidine and lysine increase free radical reactions and shorten lifespan. Radiation is a free radical generator, causing tumors in mice. This radiation effect is enhanced when unsaturated fats are added to the diet. The incidence of breast cancer in women seems to increase in proportion to the unsaturated fats in the diet. However, tumor incidence of rats fed high levels of safflower oil (an unsaturated fat) can be diminished when vitamin E (an antioxidant, free radical neutralizer) is added to their diets. Antioxidants reduced the number and severity of ultraviolet light induced cancers of the skin of mice.

Adding BHT and Santoquin to the diet of rats inhibited the accumulation of amyloid, an old age pigment—thought to be caused by the oxidative degeneration of connective tissue protein. Rats fed a form of vitamin E in a diet with unsaturated safflower oil did better on learning tests than those without vitamin E. (The frequency of judgement errors in a maze was in proportion to the concentration of safflower oil in the diet). The humoral (bone marrow, B cell) and cell mediated (thymus, T cell) immune response declined more slowly with age for those mice with Santoquin or vitamin E added to their food. BHT and 2-MEA were also effective. Serum copper levels increase with age while the mercaptans decrease (mercaptans are naturally occurring free radical scavengers). Cancer patients have elevated copper levels.

Injecting tumors with BCG, a tuberculosis vaccine, stimulates a cancer patient's immune system, thereby increasing resistance to cancer.[1] Foreign substances such

---

1. Stockton, W., A new clue in the cancer mystery, The New York Times Magazine, April 2, 1978, 18

as viruses and bacteria enter the body; lymphocytes detect the invaders who carry unique biochemical signs called antigens. The question is, do cancer cells have antigens that the immune system cannot recognize as foreign or do cancer cells flood the body with antigens, overwhelming and tying up the immune surveillance system. Or is it that small numbers of cancer cells aren't seen (their antigens are weak) or can they mask or lose their antigens.

Chemo-therapy kills cancer cells and the immune system indiscriminately. A certain illogic is at work here. What we need is something more specific, to get at the core of the mechanism: why are cancer cells not recognized as foreign and hence allowed to take hold and proliferate. The proteins possessing the ability to react with antigens are called antibodies[1]. Some T lymphocytes respond as whole cells (cell mediated)—as contrasted with B cell antibody responses (antibody mediated). With age, T cells proliferate more slowly and their numbers decline. Antibody production, indicative of B cell activity also declines.

Why do the cells lose vitality? Why does the thymus shrink? What agent induces these changes? Is it the free radical? The superoxide free radical, and the hydroxyl free radical are too reactive to be tolerated with impunity within the living system, that we know.[2] The superoxide free radical is eliminated by SOD (superoxide dismutase). In vivo SOD's have been isolated for only a decade.

The superoxide free radical is made by numerous chemical avenues in the respiring cell where SOD is fortuitously also present. Superoxide free radicals can inactivate viruses, induce lipid peroxidation (excess oxidation), damage cell membranes and killer cells yet that is not the worst of it. Superoxide is the precursor of the hydroxyl free radical, a more potent oxidant. The iron and manganese forms of SOD are found in bacteria.

---

1. Changes, Research on Aging and the Aged, D HEW publication 120 (NIH) 78-85
2. Fridovich, I., The biology of oxygen radicals, Science, Vol. 201, Sept. 8, 1978, 875-880.

Yeast, chicken livers and pig heart contain the manganese SOD in their mitochondria. Elevated levels of SOD correlate well with enhanced resistance to hyperbaric oxygen toxicity (high pressures and concentrations of oxygen). We know the presence of oxygen increases the lethality of ionizing radiation. Some reports suggest that SOD protects against this milieu and its damage to DNA, viruses and even whole mice. SOD injected as long as one hour after x-radiation of mice diminishes the lethality. It may be useful as an anti-inflammation agent by protecting against superoxide free radical damage to the synovial fluids that act as lubricating agents in the body. Thus are planted the seeds for the future claim of a new wonder drug. Time will tell, won't it, whether superoxide dismutase (SOD) and other now seemingly recondite materials will capture the imagination of the public. Superoxide may play a role in the initiation of certain cancers.[1]. SOD and another enzyme, catalase, together protect chromosomes against breakage when exposed to a radiation environment. Irradiation also produces the hydroxyl free radical which can attack cell membranes. Intravenus administration of SOD not only protects whole mice from the lethal effects of radiation but also the bone marrow cells within the animals. Externally applied SOD saves mouse skin cells from radiation moldering. Conversely, with irradiation, the SOD levels in lungs, thyroid, thymus and spleen are reduced. Should SOD levels be too low, extensive damage to cellular membrane structures could be expected. Bovine SOD is apparently non-toxic, anti-inflammatory, and effective in treating rheumatoid arthritis and joint diseases such as osteoarthritis. There may be a connection between SOD levels and longevity. Is SOD to be the rejuvenating elixer we have sought throughout our history?

The ancient Egyptians looked for such an elixir.[2] In

---

1. Michelson, A.M., Biological aspects of superoxide dismutase, in Frontiers in Physicochemical Biology, B. Pullman, editor, Academic Press, New York, 1978
2. Wallace, D.J., The biology of aging, 1976, an overview, J. Amer. Geriatrics Society, Vol. XXV, No. 3, March, 1977, 104-111

pre-biblical times the Chinese saw aging intermeshed with lifestyle (Yin and Yang). Hindus believed in continuous reincarnation which led to Nirvana. In the bible the 90th psalm records our lifespan as three score and ten. The Greek, Hippocrates (460-377 B.C.) said aging was caused by a decrease in body heat. Galen (130-201 A.D.) proposed changes in body humors—increased dryness and coldness—as the driving force. The philosopher Maimonides (1135-1204 A.D.) considered life predetermined. Roger Bacon (1210-1292 A.D.) wrote Cure of Old Age and Preservation of Youth in which he proposed to stop the aging process by good hygiene. Da Vinci (1452-1519) performed autopsies; Francis Bacon looked for our vital spirit. Santorio in the 1620's promulgated a very modern-sounding theory of hardening of the fibers and the progressive consolidation of earthy materials within the body. Darwin (1731-1762) linked aging to a failure to respond to the sense of irritability of the tissue (perhaps another way of referring to the immune system). Bichat (1771-1802) said aging is aging—the same process for all organs and tissue. Warthin (1866-1932) felt we lost energy. Hufeland (1762-1836) told again of a vital force. Metchnikoff (1845-1916) suggested autointoxication; we must at all costs prevent intestinal putrification. Brown-Sequard (1817-1894) injected animal (testicular) extracts into his own body at age 72. It was no help. Durang and Fardel in 1854 encyclopedically described changes in the body with age. Charcot (1825-1893) in the 1860's applied physiological principles and tests to study the changes. Canstatt showed cells die and are not replaced. Minot at the turn of the century studied mortality rates, following in the tradition of Gompertz (1779-1865). Kohn in 1963 said if cancer could be cured, lifespan could be extended by 3 years; stop cancer and cardiovascular diseases and we can add 10 to 15 years to reach an average longevity of 90 years. Comfort reported on the Third World peoples: the same percentage of them live to be 90 as in the Western countries, implying that our ultimate lifespan, the maximum potential, is a human characteristic independent of culture.

The maximum survival of humans is estimated to be around 115 years; the maximum doubling potential of our cells seems to be about 50 times. Consider the relationship between the two: a mouse, 3 years lifespan, 12 doublings; chickens, 30 years, 25 doublings; Galapogos tortoise, 200 years, 140 doublings.[1] Is our ultimate lifespan reflected in the doubling capacity of our cells (for those cells capable of dividing)? Is there another circumscribing factor, such as the accumulation of metabolic detritus, lipofuscin, which can be used as a benchmark? We know lipofuscin is found in the cytoplasm of the cells in the brain, muscle, myocardium, adrenal cortex, testis, ovaries, liver and kidney. Centrophenoxine (Helfergin) is capable of stimulating the metabolism of nerve cells and is able to cause lipofuscin to disappear from nerve cells and the myocardium.[2] Animals treated with centrophenoxine lived longer than a control group and had a better learning capacity. One part of centrophenoxine is a precursor of acetylcholine which comes from choline, a neurotransmitter. Should we combine centrophenoxine and SOD therapies? Would we get a synergistic effect? We know that 80 percent of the superoxide free radical in the heart is trapped by SOD.[3] The remaining 20 percent reacts with membranes, inflicting its biochemical hurts.

And how does this square with the increasing inability of cells with age to mount a graft. And T cells which are less capable of proliferating. There is a demonstrable decline in B and T cell function (T cell deficiency promotes autoantibody responses).[4] B cells secrete antibodies. They recognize free antigens and bind them to their membranes. T cells coming into the blood

---

1. Goldstein, S., W. Reichel, Physiological and biological aspects of aging, in Clinical aspects of aging, W. Reichel, editor, Williams & Wilkins, Baltimore, 1979
2. Nagy, I., A membrane hypothesis of aging, J. Theoretical Biology, Vol. 75, 1978, 189-195
3. Mays, L., Editor, Age News, American Aging Association, Vol. 9, Summer, 1979
4. Meredith, P.J., R.L. Walford, Autoimmune, histocompatibility and aging, Mechanisms of Aging and Development, Vol. 9, 1979, 61-77

from the thymus attack virus infected cells; in the presence of antigens the T cells enlarge within a few hours, produce RNA, DNA synthesis begins and results in antibody secretion.[1] After the antigen has been neutralized and digested, the activated T cells return to their former inactive state but now in larger numbers. The persistence of these newly formed T cells created by their clonal expansion forms the basis of immunological memory. Malignant cells often become antigenic to their host but sometimes, somehow, the cancer cells slip through or are impervious to our immune system. In chemotherapy we administer chemicals which are essentially suppressors of the immune system; quite possibly there could be new malignancies as a result of the treatment. We find more incidences of cancer in persons with deficient immune states, such as transplant recipients (who have received immune suppressant therapy).[2]

Normally the mortality rate is high for chickens exposed to the virulent Newcastle disease virus. BHT, a free radical scavenger when used in the chicken's diet, moderated this lethality. In high concentrations BHT was toxic in some cases, yet it also did protect chickens against the carcinogenic effects of certain chemicals and did increase lifespan in mice. The infectivity of the human herpes simplex virus is reduced in vitro (in laboratory glassware experiments, outside the body) after chickens were exposed to BHT.[3] Free radical neutralizers (antioxidants) such as BHT are known to enhance the immune response in mice. Vitamin E, in the same family, significantly improved humoral (B cell) responses whereas cell mediated (T cell) responses were best ameliorated with Santoquin. Also effective were 2-MEA and sodium hypo-

---

1. Talmadge, D.W., Recognition and memory in the cells of the immune system, American Scientist, Vol. 67, March-April, 1979, 173-178
2. Kent, S., What is the relationship of cancer to aging?, Geriatrics, November, 1977, 113-122
3. Brugh, M., Butylated hydroxytoluene protects chickens exposed to Newcastle disease virus, Science, Vol. 197, Sept. 23, 1977, 1291-2

phosphate.[1] But where is the biological clock which governs our lives?[2] Hayflick removed the nucleus from the cell cytoplasm of both old and young cells. He placed the old nucleus in the cytoplasm of young cells and found the young cells then doubled according to the older cell's lifespan potential. Conversely, a young nucleus in old cytoplasm yields a doubling and hence living capacity controlled by the young nucleus. Aging cells lose their ability to degrade protein and become "clogged" with unnecessary protein according to Gershon. In rats, mice and nematodes, enzymes (including SOD) lose 30 to 70 percent of their activity with age. Maites focused on the loss of reproductive capacity and imputed this loss to a deficiency of amines such as dopamine in the hypothalamus. Ovulation in old female rats can be induced by epinephrine, from a class of chemicals called catecholamines produced in the hypothalamus. L-dopa, a precursor of dopamine, had the same effect. Production of epinephrine and L-dopa is greater in the young than the old. But the blood of older rats contains large amounts of prolactin, a pituitary hormone which may cause pituitary and mammary tumors. Goldstein introduced calf thymosin into cancer patients and youngsters with deficient immune defenses and was able to restore T cell immune function—without side effects. Treated with thymosin, 20 immune deficient children were protected from chickenpox. Makinodan injected T cells from young into old mice; T cell activity was boosted to youthful levels for up to six months. Old mice with T cells from young mice, exposed to a vaccine against typhus, could withstand 100 times the lethal doses of the disease agent as compared to old mice with their own T cells. It would seem the next stage of this research should focus on ways to store these cells, the youthful T cells, so that they could be immediately available when needed.

---

1. Harman, D., M.L. Hendrick, D.E. Eddy, Free radical theory of aging: Effect of free radical reaction inhibitors on the immune response, J. Amer. Geriatrics Society, Vol. XXV, Sept. 1977, 400-407
2. Anonymous, Chemical changes caused by aging discovered, Chem. & Eng. News, Dec. 19, 1977, 16-18

Is aging therefore a result of alterations in the immune system or the thyroid energy generation system or errors in brain signals, or what? And are these changes caused by the onslaught of free radicals or do we first wear out, or are we programmed by some sort of rate of living constraint? Is the aging program within the cells as Hayflick proposes? And why does hydrocortisone increase the doubling potential of cells by 30 to 40 percent?[1] And what about underfeeding? Does it preserve the immune system beyond its normal expectation?[2] Early life underfeeding tampers with the rate and timing of thymus growth and involution after puberty; also core body temperature of animals is lowered. Caloric and amino acid (tryptophan) restriction affect pituitary structure and brain monoamine levels in rats in ways which ward off the stasis of old age. Put ovaries from old rats in the young and the ovaries begin cycling. Conversely, young ovaries in old rats: everything ceases.[3] Seventy percent of an old rat's liver can be removed and it will regenerate; the new tissue is old and responds weakly to glucose. Even though we've achieved regeneration of the liver, the DNA coding is sensitive to the fact that it is an old system giving the orders. Is it Denkla's death hormone in the pituitary or Hayflick's clock in the nucleus? Hypothyroidism in younger animals and people mimics premature aging, consistent with our observation that in old age thyroxine has increasing difficulty entering our cells and energizing them; we are more susceptible to infection because of diminished vitality. In the 1890's thyroxine was prescribed for humans with indolent thyroids.[4] The reversals were dramatic: wrinkles disappeared, grey hair turned black, brown or blond

---

1. Grove, G.L., V.J. Cristofalo, Characterization of the cell cycle of cultured human diploid cells, J. Cell Physiology, Vol. 90, 1976, 415-422
2. Weindruck, R.H., J.A. Kristie, K.D. Cheney, R.L. Walford, Influences of controlled dietary restriction on immunologic function and aging, Fed. Proc., Vol. 38, 1979, 2007-2016
3. Sullivan, W., Science seeks an end to the miseries of aging, New York Times, Nov. 16, 1975
4. Rosenfeld, A., Are we programmed to die? Saturday Review, Oct. 2, 1970, 10-17

again; resistance to disease returned to normal. However, for those who were just old, with normal thyroid function, the treatment didn't work. Indeed with high treatment levels of thyroxine there were some deaths and this procedure was stopped.

Not everyone believes in a deterministic approach to aging. Some favor a stochastic philosophy which says life is a series of events governed by the laws of probability. By virtue of cells and molecules bumping into each other, changes occur; changes leading to free radicals, wear and tear, errors in the synthesis of DNA, deviant brain function and weakened immune vitality. The avataristic commitment theory deals with the possibility that when cells double, what is produced is not two identical, equally youthful daughter cells, but two different daughter cells: one able to continue to proliferate (uncommitted) and the other older and unable to do this and hence committed to death. Other stochastic theories relate to: the survival curve analysis[1] and cell division as a diluter of its essence.[2,3] These theories have some utility in attempting to understand why epithelial cells of mouse duodenum and small intestine have a turnover rate of two days, parenchymal cells of the liver are replaced in 160 to 400 days, nerve and muscle cells live for 1000 days and never divide. In the rat and mouse liver, parenchymal cells (60 percent of the liver) are replaced at the rate of one per 20,000 each 24 hour period.[4]

Bee stings or ointments containing bee venom somehow are helpful in stimulating the immune system[5] and are used in the treatment of rheumatism, infectious

---

1. Woodbury, M.A., K.G. Manton, A random-walk model of human mortality and aging, Theoret. Population Biology, 1977, 37-48
2. Hirsch, H.R., The waste-product theory of aging: waste dilution by cell division, Mech. of Aging and Development, Vol. 8, 1978, 51-62
3. Hirsch, H.R., The dynamics of repetitive cell division, Mech. of Aging and Development, Vol. 6, 1977, 319-322
4. Gahan, P.B., Increased levels of euploidy as a strategy against rapid aging in diploid mammalian systems, Exp. Geront, Vol. 12, 1977, 133-136
5. Vick, J.A., W. Shipman, G.B. Warren, C. Mraz, R. Brooks, Studies of the venom of the honey bee, Report from the Office of the Surgeon General, Toxicon 10, 1972, 6

polyarthritis, spondyl-arthritis deformans, trophic ulcers, asthma, migraine. The venom can be delivered topically in oily or aqueous solution or by subcutaneous injection. Considerable swelling and inflammation results, without fatalities. It's a four-week treatment; children seem to respond most quickly. Controversial? Certainly, but if we strip away the bizarre aspects—using live bees as the vector—what is apparently happening is nothing more complicated than a stimulation of the immune system. And it seems to work, not only for some old patients but also for a 15 year old girl who suffered from precocious or premature aging. She had low levels of active T cells (the total count of T cells was also depressed) and had a family history of cancer.[1] Can we use bee sting therapy to treat lupus erythematosis, an autoimmune disease?[2]

The confluence of nutrition, lifespan and free radicals is an exciting, albeit unproved concept. There are no shortages of "magical" diets, synthesized for maximum effect on longevity. You can increase lifespan for mice and guinea pigs by adding the amino acid cysteine to the diet, or a combination of thiazolidinecarboxylic acid and folic acid (all containing sulfur and hydrogen atoms chemically bound). Passwater and Welker[3] theorized that antioxidants (free radical scavengers) in the diet could add 5 to 10 years to our lifespan, sulfhydryl compounds (containing sulfur) which afford radiation protection and are free radical scavengers could add another 2 to 5 years and protein missynthesis correctors (containing selenium) could contribute 5 to 10 additional years. Taken together in one diet, assuming the three factors act synergistically, we may hope for, according to Passer and Welker, an extra 30 to 40 years of longevity. The

---

1. Schuman, S.H., N.N. Fudenberg, J.M. Goust, R. Jorgenson, T-cells, precocious aging and familial neoplasia, Gerontology, Vol. 24, 1978, 266-275
2. Horowitz, S., W. Borcherding, A.V. Moorthy, R. Chesney, H. Schulte-Wasserman, R. Hong, A. Goldstein, Induction of suppressor T cells in systemic lupus erythematosis by thymidin and cultured thymic epithelium, Science, Vol. 197, Sept. 2, 1977, 999-1001
3. Passwater, R.A., P.A. Welker, Human aging research, American Laboratory, May, 1971, 21-26

sulfhydryl compounds taken in conjunction with vitamin E are supposed to increase our tolerance to selenium which is supposed to be able to control the errors of DNA production of protein. Foods containing selenium include tuna, herring, menhadden, anchovette, brewers yeast, wheat germ, bran, broccoli, onions, cabbage and tomatoes. Foods high in sulfur amino acids are eggs, cabbage, muscle meats, wheat germ oil, leafy vegetables, fish, whole wheat, vegetable oils.

Oxygen uptake by the blood in the lungs is down from 4 liters per minute at 20 years of age to 1.5 liters per minute at 75 years. No wonder old folks don't function as well as before. And why are there these changes in brain function: increased nighttime awakenings; decreased length of periods of deep sleep; loss of short term memory; and depression.[1] Does it have any relation to the observation that our neurons accumulate lipofuscin, that there is a loss in the brain of dendrite and synaptic connections, the transporters of signals? We measure a decrease with age of dopamine in the corpus striatum portion of the brain. The neurotransmitters dopamine, norepinephrine and serotonin affect the hypothalamus; the hormones from the hypothalamus cause the release of CAMP, an activator of cell metabolism and the RNA which carries the protein synthesis messages. Aging is associated with smaller concentrations of neurotransmitters such as dopamine, acetylcholine and gamma-amino butyric acid (GABA) in the brain and the hypothalamus. In rats, a diet low in the amino acid tryptophan slows growth and development, delays reproductive functions.

Feeding L-dopa extends life for mice. Iproniazide reinitiates estrous cyclicity in old rats and seems to rejuvenate them in general. Makinodan and Albright[2] tested 2-MEA on immune function and found it restored old rats to a more youthful level.

---

1. Timaras, P.S., Biological perspectives on aging, American Scientist, Vol. 61, Sept.-Oct., 1978, 605-613
2. Makinodan, T., J.W. Albright, Restoration of impaired immune function in aging animals, Mech. Aging and Development, Vol. 10, 1979, 325-340

Ancient Egyptians ate garlic to ward off death. The alchemists of China prescribed gold and mercury to do the same. We have eaten mandrake roots and allowed ourselves to contact fever blisters, to get monkey gland transplants, to inject procaine into our blood—all in the elusive search for good health and rejuvenation. Are we programmed to self-destruct with time, a basically pessimistic theory of aging? Are there errors constantly cropping up, or as in the masochist's dream do we misidentify ourselves, see our reflection as a foreign invader—and attack and attack and attack until there is nothing left to recognize? Are the chemical bridges of collagen and other structural materials altered with age, causing us to function dolorously—increasingly so until we are sufficiently weakened and die? Or do we in living, desecrate our living edifice with biological detritus? We search and research the means for survival, from vitamins E and C, to free radicals, to bacteria which can eat old collagen, to thymosin and its effect on the immune system, to centrophenoxine to stimulate the hypothalamus, to dopamine for proper brain function and even to starvation for a slower growth rate. All in the name of survival.

We have found tumors linked with prolactin in old pituitaries in remarkable frequency[1] and we wonder what that means. We know that free radicals are produced during cell respiration, during irradiation damage and from environmental pollutants such as ozone.[2] Free radicals cause excessive oxidation of lipids and cell membrane damage and accumulation of aging pigments. Superoxide dismutase (SOD), glutathione peroxidase, vitamin E, vitamin C and selenium are of importance as free radical neutralizers and proscribers of excess lipid oxidation, yet the levels of vitamin C, selenium and mercaptans appear to decline as we age. And isn't that a pity?

---

1. Kovacs, K., N. Ryan, E. Horvath, W. Singer, C. Ezrin, Pituitary adenomas in old age, J. Gerontology, Vol. 35, No. 1, 1980, 16-22
2. Leibovitz, B.E., B.V. Siegel, Aspects of free radical reactions in biological systems aging, J. Gerontology, Vol. 35, No. 1, 1980, 45-56

Chapter 4

Death In Conclusion

Rotting Ginsberg, I stared in the mirror naked today
I noticed the old skull, I'm getting balder
my pate gleams in the kitchen light under thin hair
like the skull of some monk in old catacombs lighted by
a guard with flashlight
followed by a mob of tourists
so there is death

What happens when the death gong hits rotting Ginsberg
    on the head
what universe do I enter
death death death death death the cat's at rest
are we ever free of—rotting Ginsberg
Then let it decay, thank God I know
thank who
thank who
Thank you, O lord, beyond my eye
the path must lead somewhere
the path
the path.
           From MESCALINE by Alan Ginsberg

Dear Michael:
    When will you realize that you are not immortal, that you too, as everyone else who was ever born, will die. And what a crashingly sober thought, what a depressing thought, to realize that you will walk the earth, love your parents and your house and wife and children and the sunset and so many other natural and artificial objects, animate and inanimate, but this love, the experiences, the help you render, that pleasure obtained, all will end after seventy, eighty or one-hundred years. Why go on at all, you will ask, on that day when you come to understand the realities of being moribund. Why not join the hedonists

and screw everyone. Let's enjoy ourselves. Eat everything you like and don't bother with the rest. Go to bed with anyone who'll please you and don't worry about marriage, children, religion, morality, and politics. Enjoy. Enjoy. And perhaps, Michael, you will succumb. Don't build bridges, don't bother with linkages, who cares about the future? Why plan for our children? Why care whether institutions live or die? I won't be around to see it so who the hell thinks about the future?

Michael, what is death? Do you believe that I shall die and soon thereafter we shall see each other again and play the same roles as before: I, the daddy, and you, the little boy—son. Or is death the end, the irrevokable, unalterable cessation of breathing, thinking and being. Are we alive because of the intermingling of corporeal, ethereal and esthetic senses? It is indeed difficult to face the possibility that death is the end, that death is the only reality and everything else is the illusion. No one lives in a vacuum, for nothing exists in a vacuum. If there were no one else, I would be of no consequence. If there is no one to hear me, does it matter if I talk? Who cares what I think, if thinking doesn't affect you. I live every day; I talk and play and learn. But, Michael, I can feel death coming. It is written in many ways. Not only by the apparent loss of physical prowess, not only by altered appearances which we can recite, but as exactly and relentlessly as the most perfect mathematical formula. I see it by the maturing of my human relationships. In our youth, in our ascendency, these relationships are budding and building, becoming more intermeshed with others. The life's forces form intersecting patterns which are surely definable and may be quantitatively described. Michael, we reach our peak when our tentacles of human associations are maximized. Then we decline, slowly from this zenith, and more rapidly, in our later years, as the binding tentacles wither and the complexities unravel. We tend towards simpler, fewer relationships as parents die, children grow and move away and friendships recede. To be sure, new growths occur, and fresh connections develop, but these new strands are less vital, less viable and surely less fertile. So life and death can be traced out. And I am conscious of the beginning of the end for me. My father is dead, my mother, your grandmother, is very old now. Your mother's father and mother are also in the late mature phase. It is possible that by your fifteenth birthday you shall no longer be able to visit your grandma where you now have such happy times. Other relationships of mine are likewise beginning to fade at an accelerated rate—or so it seems.

Michael, when I am fifty, it is likely that I shall be head of the family: both sides of the family—and hence shall assume the stance of the elder. It is a nervous thought, Michael, since I have never considered myself in this light before. My hair, which is thinning on top may be even less dense at fifty and I expect a bit greyer where it remains. I am pleased with my physical condition now, Michael, content with the degree of muscle tone and my weight. Michael, at fifty will I be as able physically as now? I shall strive for this but we know that something must be lost sooner or later. There is no denying the relentless loss of physical prowess with age. Though I take vitamin C, E, one-a-day vitamins and zinc, I am troubled these days by a return to the pattern of having too many colds, which was the bane of my youth in New York. I am beginning to worry as each winter it seems as if the severity of the malady intensifies. Am I losing my vitality and hence my resistance to disease or is it simply that I am seeing your virulent virus germs? We shall see where this leads, won't we? At least I am aware of the trends and the dangers.

As far as I can determine, my mental abilities are as yet unimpaired. Assuming enough blood and oxygen reach my brain and I get sufficient exercise, I expect to suffer no significant losses for awhile. But who knows whether a gradual loss of body health won't lead to a weakened mental condition? This is an unknown factor in the aging process. We wish desperately that the mind will not dull, that senility does not overtake us. But it happens to so many and we may conclude that the odds are not in our favor. Michael, it is now understood that those who are stimulated steadily by job and play, who maintain that marvelous tension of life, who are inquiring by nature, are not easily hobbled by senility. Since I take pride in my inquiring mind and do the correct things, I do not expect to become senile—unless I suffer a major upset in my homeostasis.

It is difficult to picture yourself as old. What will I look like at seventy? Probably a good deal like my father. By then muscle mass will be wasted so we shall be able to see folds of useless flesh. I expect I will be as thin as was my father. The minor hurts, such as back pains or pulled muscles we incur now—and recover from—become more serious at seventy and we do not shake them off so readily. If my colds persist into my seventies, then shall pneumonia be lurking around the corner? At seventy, pneumonia is very serious indeed. Cancer probably will be no threat since it doesn't run in our family and I don't smoke. Michael, if my prognosis is correct, my old age will find me constantly in danger of respiratory diseases and with it, the steady weakening of age-diminished lung function. I may die one day in my seventies or later, of what the doctors will diagnose as pneumonia, but the cause of death will actually be old age. I hope to be vigorous to the end for I intend to exercise and be stimulated and interested in my ambience.

What if we could live forever. Michael, what is forever? What is infinity? Do you know? You can count fairly well, now, Michael. You are able to recite one, two three,...twenty, twenty-one,...ninety-nine, one-hundred. And then you begin again. You love to count, marveling as you go up the ladder at the order of things while soaking up the praise exuded by parents and friends. But what happens as we count higher, up to one-million, one-billion, one-trillion, one-thousand-trillion? Michael, I can always add one more to whatever number your counting concludes with, so you see there is really no end to your counting. To put it another way, the end is at infinity, which is an imaginary concept and a mathematical convenience. How do you reach infinity?

You and I, Michael, are composed of billions of cells. We are the summed total of all these cells and collectively we can talk and think and touch. We see and can be seen, though the single cell may be invisible to our eyes. Growing in us and on us are smaller bacteria. Attached to and inside the bacteria are yet smaller things called viruses which are thought to be the smallest "living" creatures. But viruses are composed of molecules which give them their character. These molecules are built up by combining smaller units called atoms. Atoms are collections of electrons, neutrons, protons and still smaller bits and pieces of matter and energy. And what are the electrons, neutrons and protons composed of? Probably energy, sheer ethereal stuff which may travel in waves.

Having gone down the scale, from you and me to the atoms and to floating packets of energy, Michael, let's go up the ladder. We rest on a piece of land called earth, which is a sphere rotating and orbiting in a galaxy of billions of other gigantic particles in the Milky Way. And beyond our universe there must be more galaxies and doesn't it logically follow that we in our world must be part of a larger system of stars and planets? And can't we expect that this larger system is really a subunit of a still greater, more complicated operation?

And where does it end? At infinity, of course. But where is it? And who does the counting of the systems which lead to infinity? Can we ever find the answer to the question? Michael, is this why we believe in God?

Michael, looking up and down the scale of things, down to the smallest, invisible waves, up to the stars and infinity, does all our discussion of living and dying have a new perspective? We live and die as part of a grand design, as do our body cells and the stars. We shall evolve, Michael, and who knows towards what? Eventually, perhaps in a million years, our brains may be so highly developed that human communication will require only brain waves and not involve the other senses. We'll receive each other's signals without corporeal intervention. In other words we will not need our bodies. Thus our bodies will wither and at some point in the future we shall be unshackled from the tangible, shuck off the skin, bones and blood and float through space as wave packets of intelligence. And then, Michael, how shall you define life and death? Will it be a better life? Surely it will be different and unrelated to our present frame of reference. Is it possible that already we are experiencing on earth the intervention of these other life forces? Who is to say that it is not possible for these alien explorers to travel through the universe and finding us on earth, interject themselves into our bodies and minds and thus influence our history? Do you allow this possibility, Michael? Do you accept infinity? I believe, and therefore pose these questions for you. And from these questions, Michael, is derived my morality and mortality.

I know I am but an infinitesimal cog in a larger, infinite order of things. I am governed by the laws of probability and some other moral forces which guide my actions. I love and play and learn because I enjoy the experience and it proves helpful to my fellow cogs who are, on my level, called human beings. Someone up there is watching us, and I do my part to make our system work. This means trying to be considerate, honest, constructive and loving. I am no saint; I suffer the same lusts as others. I am jealous of my right to work for the betterment of my immediate family and the family of man. Through all of this, I am constantly aware of the larger scheme of things and therefore I sometimes become a bit detached from the usual daily thoughts and pressures. Michael, we do not die alone, for around us, above us, on us and within us are dependent folks, whether they be relatives, friends, bacteria on our skin, parasites and viruses in our blood or others once removed. We shall be born, live and die, and in being, alter the universe. The march towards infinity will be affected ever so slightly. The record of my existence adds to this progression. Very few humans will be aware of my history. But I know, Michael, and by knowing I endeavor to construct a meaningful record.

Chapter 5

My Aged Father

Strange now to think of you, gone without corsets and eyes, while
  I walk on the sunny pavement of Greenwich Village
downtown Manhattan, clear winter noon, and I've been up
  all night, talking, talking, reading the Kaddish aloud,
  listening to Ray Charles blues about blind on the
  phonograph
the rhythm the rhythm—and your memory in my head three
  years after—and read Adonais' last triumphant stanzas
  aloud—wept, realizing how we suffer
And how Death is that remedy all singers dream of, sing,
  remember, prophesy as in the Hebrew Anthem, or the
  Buddhist Book of Answers—and my own imagination of
  a withered leaf—at dawn
Dreaming back thru life, Your time—and mine accelerating
  toward Apocalypse,
the final moment—the flower burning in the Day—and what
  comes after.
from KADDISH by Alan Ginsberg

    My father died three days ago. Michael, he was your grandpa, your father's father and you hardly knew him. How could you? Your life has spanned only four years but this is only a small fraction of grandpa's seventy-eight. And now he is dead, succumbing finally to the ravages of tobacco smoke, emphysema, hardening of the arteries, diminished blood flow to the brain—and old age. When he died he was shriveled and shrunken at eighty-five pounds, worn out from the pain of his illness and crying for death. The inhuman piece-work tailoring he did throughout his life for the Amalgamated Clothing Workers Union had taken its toll. Michael, he was paid by the number of finished pieces he registered at week's end, and this beautifully efficient method of production made a slave of him, ruined his nerves and sapped his energy. Grandpa died because his body was used up.

And now as we, my father's family, sit in mourning, I think of my father. Michael, I think of you also for I didn't know my father very well—and I wonder if upon my own death, when you recapitulate and reenact my ritual, will you also say of me: I hardly knew my father. I feel fine, Michael. There are no aches and pains which limit my functions. I eat well, have physical vigor and enjoy a full sex life. But the signs are there, Michael, for those who wish to look: the loss of hair on the head, grey ones sprouting where before only a field of black existed and brown-pigmented spots on the skin. You look upon me as eternally youthful, Michael, you cannot conceive of death for me because daddys don't die. But I shall die, Michael, as we all shall die, but I cannot tell you this. I shall not remain eternally the one-hundred years of age you ascribe to me, nor will your mother remain at twenty. I have long ceased to grow, though you think of me as getting bigger and bigger. Adam's daddy is not older than I because he is taller, but you enjoy this illusion and why should I try to change your beliefs. Michael, you ask me whether you will die and I am troubled in searching for an answer. I know you will die eventually, but should I tell you this. You tell me very smugly that grandpa smoked and therefore got old and died because he got old. So if you do not smoke, you reason you will not get old and hence will not die. A sophisticated logical chain for a four-year-old to construct, Michael. There is time for you to learn the truth.

Michael, my father came as a youth from Hungary to New York in a manner unknown to me, lived on the lower East Side of Manhattan as those before him did and gravitated to the East New York section of Brooklyn as the wave of immigrants swelled past Manhattan into the hinterlands. Your grandpa, Michael, my father, always seemed to me to be the stereotype of the Jewish immigrant, arriving with an imperfect knowledge of the old language, a semi-skilled means for earning a living in the new country, a sense of religion (but no fanaticism) and a will to survive. Through the years he learned to read

English haltingly but acceptably (though he preferred to read the Yiddish papers), never lost his "Jewish" accent when he spoke "American", found a garment center job which he clung to for survival and married a Rumanian girl who was to become my mother, your grandma. Michael, the early photographs of my father show a fire in the eyes which he lost only in his penultimate days. He was proud, stubborn and masculine; all these traits I surmise, Michael, for I really didn't know him until the decade before his death when he was retired and into the terminal phase of his life and I was established in mine and confident of my station.

I have no vivid recollections of my father as a young man, only a vague sense of his strong presence in the house, though he was away at work for an extended period each day. Even his mature years evoke blurred images, for our household was run by your grandma, who ruled benevolently. My father was gone much of the time and so was I, out on the streets, or in the candy stores, or in school. Michael, you must know me better than I knew your grandpa. He was a man, of flesh and blood who now is dead and ready to be buried. Who will remember him? What were his accomplishments? What will live on afterward, with his imprint? Why was he born? Of what consequence was his life?

My father retired into oblivion, becoming a household pet where previously he enjoyed the prestige as leader of the pride. With no planning for retirement, with no hobbies which could command his attention, with no skills adaptable to New York City cliff dwelling, with a lifetime of specialized work yielding a sum total of zero upon retirement, your grandpa and grandma encountered the irresistable forces of senility and impending death as grandpa's life energy ebbed steadily and monotonically. The tiger was down. What do I remember best of my father? Michael, I recall the sadness and humiliation of old age as he sensed his powers slipping away. But for one brief period, he endeavored to reverse the process by returning to work part time. By all accounts the resumption of his old tailoring trade rejuvenated his powers, lifted his spirits and introduced hope into the household. And then, Michael, our government imposed itself to tell this old man he should act his age. Do not work, old man, they said. In your retirement you must sit at home and rock. So they added up his earnings, declared that he had accumulated too much in wages and subtracted the excess from his sacred social security benefits. That will teach you, old man, don't do it again or we shall deal with you more severely. My father cried, he was diminished by the government he loved, he was shamed into believing that he had done something criminal. He still could sew at home, fixing this, patching that, occasionally coordinating his design and manual skills in the synthesis of an overcoat or a pair of trousers. But he was on the human garbage heap and knew it. My father now understood the verity of old age, that no matter what medicines were taken, you never could feel "one-hundred percent". Life was indeed irreversible and he would soon die.

Chapter 6
Losses With Age

Talk of aging and the finiteness of life seems to become peculiarly a battle of science versus sociology, as we attempt to generate an unemotional ambience for our discussion. In the audiences there is a certain fear—and some resentment. Don't tell me about getting old. Don't tell me that I may reach my peak at age 40 if I am a writer or scientist, or that age 30 to 35 is my zenith if I am an athlete.[1] I won't hear of it. I don't wish to die. But the questions must be asked. How old are you? How do you know how old you are? Look about you. Who is older? How do you know this?

We know there is a variability of lifespan in us and animals and even trees: that a Douglas Fir has different age brackets from teenage puberty to old-age senility which in the fir begins around 160 years of age. As we first raise the question, Must We Die?, we note that U.S. women apparently live longer than U.S. men.

Must we die? Probably. Can we extend life or take steps to make our old age more pleasant and healthy? Yes, we can, if you will accept that in rats you may limit the calorie intake of the young and find a diminished rate of generation of neoplasms in the old rats. Chronically restricted diets for young rats resulted in about one-half the number of multiple tumors in these rats. For every ten percent reduction of body weight, there seems to be in these rats a 13.5 percent gain in life expectancy. Such a dietary regimen maintained a relatively short period early in life produced long-lasting effects later. However, for older rats, severe dietary restriction decreased lifespan. So, there are indeed things we can do for the rats to

---

1. Hershey, D., Lifespan and factors affecting it, Thomas, Springfield, 1974.

affect lifespan. Do these data extrapolate to humans? Probably. Is the analogy exact? Who knows?

To keep alert and well, it is known now that we should exercise and this may lower the resting heart rate, increase maximum physiological work capacity and maximum oxygen uptake. Workouts on a bicycle reduce heart rate and systolic blood pressure. Being in good physical condition means greater utilization of oxygen in muscle tissue regardless of age. Middle-aged men who participated in calisthenics, swimming or jogging for ten weeks showed a decrease in heart rate before and after these exercise programs. Calisthenics, swimming or jogging affects the cardiorespiratory system in a way that recommends this activity to all of us, particularly the middle-aged and elderly. However, the average lifespan of athletes is the same as the general population though college graduates live longer than others. Of the athletes, football players had the shortest lifespan, then in order of increasing lifespan there are the boxers, basketball players, and track and field performers who had the longest lifespan of the athletes. Men with academic honors live two years longer on the average than their college classmates. We need all the help available as we get older, for we know that there is a steady loss of physical strength with age, a loss of about 50 percent of our capacity in going from age 20 to 70. It is more difficult for the elderly to survive in working environments at elevated temperatures, as measured by accident frequency of coal miners, where the strongest of them seem to be in the 35 to 45 year age bracket. Cardiac activity, acid secretion in the stomach, maximum breathing capacity, nerve conduction velocity are all down with age, as is our sense of taste and sight. Thus, in the snowy winter we ought not walk out of our homes and commence to shovel the snow off the walk, for this wrenching stress taxes the heart and vascular system too drastically, too suddenly, and should there be a slight physiological weakness, a heart attack can result. The digestive system is not up to the challenge of large, fatty meals if you are old. As a result, the elderly may be diabetic temporarily and unable to convert their foods properly for 24 hours while the young can do the job in a few hours. More sugar is needed in coffee and tea for sweetening if you are old. The eyes yellow and the pupils dilate less and more slowly in the old, resulting in less seeing ability in marginal lighting situations. Driving at night now becomes dangerous for the old since not only are their reflexes slowed, but the headlights may not provide enough light to see by. Thus, for the old and young driving at night at the same speed, it is more likely that the old will be guilty of not seeing well enough. In the old brain, small arterioles are found to have moderately thickened walls containing an amyloid-like material (composed of albumin and other materials). The cortex or outer layer has a shrunken appearance. There is a decrease in brain cell count, a deposit of yellow-brown lipofuscin, an increase in water content in the brain, a decrease in total solids and a loss of protein and vitamin C in the old brain.

As we age it is possible to chart the symptoms of psychological stagnation, such as low esteem and a fear of competition, even fear of success. Those facing difficulties adjusting to getting old generally say time is short, too short to start another life or to try alternate roads. There is a fear of loss of self-respect for we cannot admit that what we are doing may no longer be good enough. The antidote is "successful aging", by staying in training in an intellectual and devotional sense. Successful aging usually means having a spouse or close partner living and available. In one survey of an over-65 group, 87 percent seem to be free of serious mental health problems which is good news. Yet there are some reasons for disquiet: in the over-65 population, 25 percent had physical disabilities, 90 percent seemed socially isolated, 10 to 14 percent were in severe economci straits, 21 percent were unable to care for their basic daily needs, 27 percent had transportation problems, 8 percent needed personal care services, 24 percent were in need of immediate medical services and 21 percent required coordinated services.

Sexually, the elderly seem to be better off than we imagined. The orgasm in older women is identical to that in younger women, though the orgasmic phase is reduced. Of the 250 geriatric subjects studied, over one-half of the married persons were active sexually. In the 62 to 71 year old married group, mean frequency of intercourse was twice weekly while the 72 to 81 year population had an average of three per month. At age 68, seventy percent of the men still regularly partake in sexual activity; at age 78, twenty-five percent of the men were still sexually active. But very few unmarried older women report regular sexual activity. Unavailability of a sanctioned sexual partner seems to be the chief determinent.

We cannot work as well at elevated temperatures as we used to, our tendency is to have more accidents. The strength in our muscles is diminished even though our muscle cells do not suggest the loss of function. Our reaction time is down from its peak quickness and so is our back strength. Our cardiac function diminishes steadily into old age and so does breathing capacity. There is a loss in the ability of the lungs to let air through the lung membranes. As a general rule, we can say that there is a one percent loss in function for each year of life. Stomach acid secretions drop with age so it becomes more difficult to digest those spicy hot dogs and pickles, less blood is pumped through the kidneys, the metabolic rate drops as does one's nerve conduction velocity. After age forty the human death rate doubles each successive eight year period.

As we get older we need continuous assurance or new information as we proceed in the solution of problems put before us. We reassure ourselves by repeated visual examination of the stimulus. We make more errors in translating spatial perceptions into motor performance. The input and output of information is more tightly coupled and it is harder to change the response. An error made is more difficult to correct. We are losing speed and flexibility and reserves. Memory starts to fade generally around age thirty but vocabulary comprehension scarcely changes with maturation and old folks, given enough time, can come up with the right answers in decision-making tests. Brain weight is down. There is a decline in oxygen consumption in the brain as we get older and we accumulate old age pigments around the heart and neurons of the brain. With age there is a progressive loss of taste buds in the mouth. In the young, taste buds have been found on the roof of the mouth, walls of the throat and on the central and upper parts of the tongue. No wonder foods taste so good. But by age ten these are gone and we are left with taste buds only on the front, back and sides of the tongue. Hence we put more sugar in our coffee than before.

Our eyes get yellowish with age and less transparent. We detect less violet colors. Aging artists' sense of color changes with age and they tend to use more violet. Older persons need more light to see. While driving a car, old folks see less well because they need more illumination. For every thirteen years of age, the light intensity must be doubled in order to fully see an object. It becomes important to recognize this when driving an automobile at night. Though the elderly person's eyesight may be normal, he or she still needs more light than the younger person in order to see properly. Thus if the old drive at "normal" speeds at night, there will be a tendency to overdrive the headlights. The elderly need to go at slower speeds at night. By the fifth decade of life our eyes usually need correction with convex lenses because of a loss of adaptibility of the eye lens, not being as elastic as before. We get stiffer with age, which is not news for those of us who try to stay athletic and graceful in our later years. It has to do with our connective tissue which binds and supports tendons, ligaments, skin, blood vessels, bone and teeth among other things. Thus, we must warm up more thoroughly at advanced ages, before being athletic again, while the young can begin to run and jump immediately. Because the cartilages between one bone and the next also get thinner, it has been found that by age sixty we are about one-half inch shorter than we were before. Into our old age, we shall have lost much of the fat on our bodies. We may be thirty pounds lighter at age eighty than at forty.

Radiation produces free radicals by interaction with cellular water. Cosmic radiation and other background sources also subject us to free radicals. Can this constant, ambient level of radiation produce a low level of naturally occurring mutations in a species? Are we now the result of this background radiation—and what would we look like if this were removed? In exposure experiments on animals, the results indicate that a single radiation dose of one roentgen is equivalent in humans to 5 to 10 days of extra age. Radiation also causes increased tumor generation, as if we were older than we really are. Neoplasms such as leukemia show up earlier in irradiated mice. Genetic errors are more prevalent after radiation treatment: liver cells of mice show about twice the normal number of chromosome aberrations after a life shortening dose. With radiation, lesions and degenerative diseases show up in small blood vessels and the walls of the arterioles. Small arteries are thickened with connective tissue. Whole-body irradiation experiments on mice show that the death rate is considerably accelerated by increasing levels of single dose radiation: and that the young are more sensitive to this stress. The nature of the environment during irradiation has some effect on the death rate. It appears that radiation exposure in a pure oxygen environment is deadlier than in normal air or pure nitrogen.

Chapter 7

Hey, Michael,

It's Your Daddy

You and I, Michael, have a special relationship. You are physically well-endowed, and in possession of a strong, straight and handsome body. You are strong-willed now, determined to do things your own way even if there is some breakage along the way. You have courage and mental alertness and toughness which are admirable traits when harnessed properly. As you find yourself, Michael, as you become more coordinated, as you grow older and become more physically and mentally formed, I shall rejoice in your accomplishments. In the meantime, Michael, I attempt to control your excesses, to chip away at the rough edges which need refining. You do not always appreciate this training, Michael. We do have some disagreements: "Go to your room and come out when you think you can behave properly," I say to you often. And you go, Michael, knowing that I mean it and am determined to be heeded—and also that I do it with much love in my heart for you. Nothing that happens diminishes my love for you. How often have I commanded, "Get control of yourself." "Hold it." They seem to be my favorite expressions of constraint. I have even whacked you on the behind, which you hate, but accept, as I tell you in exact terms the nature of the transgression which generated the punishment. I do all this at the time of crisis, when it must be faced. We are open, Michael, you and I, and have always been this way. You are able to soar euphorically to the highest plateaus. I delight in observing your free spirit reaching, reaching. There is no meaness in you, Michael, even when you are angry with me, for we talk, you explain, you reveal and I listen and we understand. You wear your emotions on your sleeve Michael, your face is the heralder of your innermost thoughts. You are so vulnerable against a scheming adult or older child and not surprising, they have occasionally taken advantage of you. As you grow older and wiser and more knowledgeable of the intricacies of life, some of this openness will surely disappear, Michael, but I pray there will be enough of a residue to keep you one of the beautiful people. Michael, my days are a joy because of your presence in our home, in our family.

Michael, I think about death quite a bit these days, about my own death and that of others. I am dying steadily, I can feel it. In all likelihood, from a probabilistic point of view, my life is more than half over and I now wonder what one feels at death. It is not death itself which I fear and try to avoid, rather it is the sense of loss in not being able to see you grow and mature and develop your distinct station in life. I am reasonably confident that your mother will be able to survive my absence; the insurance on my life will guarantee fiscal continuity even if I am not on the scene. But, Michael, I wish to be with you, to help guide you, to counsel with you, to experience another facet of life through your eyes and senses. Not to live again but to refresh my own experiences, having them leavened by your presence.

Death isn't lurking imminently, yet I understand fully the signs, such as when I get a feeling of heaviness in the chest after working too many hours without sleeping sufficiently. I interpret this as a warning. Surely my arteries are beginning to clog, as have the arteries of those before me. I look backward more often now, not attributing this solely to the nostalgic phase of life but mostly to the terminalis syndrome, the ultimate understanding of the finiteness of lifespan.

Michael, when I die, there will probably be a flash of pain, a short interval of panic as breathing ceases, as residual oxygen is consumed in the tissues and the brain and there is that last instinctive gasp—and then nothing. Then, Michael, you are on your own and I hope and pray you shall remember me fondly, as one who loved you, as one who was your friend as well as father. My zest for life, my enthusiasm and basic optimism, I trust is imbued in you but I have no guarantee. So I selfishly grieve for me, and am anxious for you. Will you have the strength to be happy and successful, to be able to construe a meaningful and satisfying life? I don't know and I worry.

Michael, as I consider the death of animate and inanimate things, as I contemplate my own death and reflect on the fact that I am the sum total of an almost infinite number of internal and external interactions and stresses, so I have come to see countries, my country, similarly. The United States of America has been born, is reenacting the known phases of life and will in all probability senesce and die. That which I have said about living systems, I reiterate, extending the comparison to my country and the others. We are all analogous. History is nothing more than the tracing out of the lifespans of particular species of humanity, sometimes grouped together in some recognizable set. Thus, Michael, I naturally take a longer view of internal and external politics (national and international). There is a certain programmed character to life, which seems to include cannibalism and inhumanly savage conflicts. My tolerance of things the way they are does not imply an existential or laissez-faire detachment. Though I see the world through my aging gerontologist's eye, and perhaps acknowledge too readily the rationale for the good and bad that we do, I draw the line at war. Michael, it does sometimes seem natural for us, the supposed higher form of life, to engage in merciless slaughter of our own kind. There ought to be other ways to resolve conflicts than by war, by blatant murderings (after we have been properly indoctrinated by our leaders to hate our fellow human beings whom we call the enemy). Thus, Michael, I shall not encourage you to go to war. I shall not allow you to be available, if I have any influence on you. I shall not forfeit your life and limbs, I shall not put your life in the ultimate danger simply to satisfy a short-term whim and resolve of a few men and women who are our leaders. For what purpose were they killed in Korea and Vietnam. For what holy purpose. Our enemies are now our friends and our friends soon shall be our enemies. If there is anything which ought to remain constant, it is the sanctity of life. My lifespan belongs to me; it is mine to use as I see fit and Michael, so does yours. No President has the right to demand your life for his cause.

Michael, I am saying that no one, no President, no Congress, no country has the right to require me to give my life for their cause. I may volunteer to put my life in jeopardy, given the proper circumstances, but I do not allow that Lyndon Johnson, Richard Nixon, Gerald Ford, Jimmy Carter or anyone else can force me into a life-threatening situation. Oh, how I've changed, Michael, from the World War II mentality, when the cause against the barbaric Nazis and Japanese was the New Crusade, as we defended the United States and its freedom. They threatened the entire world and who could resist the clarion call to arms. The goals were holy; we were to save mankind. So it seemed perfectly proper to be drafted and thereby be required to surrender one's life if circumstances dictated this sacrifice. Eventually the war ended, Michael, and before anyone knew what was happening, our enemies became our allies, our former allies became the ugly threat as the world turned topsy-turvy. Then the Korean War came along and our country was aligned with the United Nations and the forces for good against North Korea, Russia, China and the Communist Horde. This was the war to preserve democracy in the Far East, otherwise the "slime" would engulf all of us, our leaders told us. They exhorted us to volunteer for the armed services, but just to be sure of our commitment, our leaders offered us a forced conscription, the draft, the ensure a national effort. Who the hell really cared about Korea, who believed in the domino theory? Why were we dying out there? For freedom? Michael, when the propaganda was stripped from the camouflaged words of our diplomats, there was the truth for all to see. The North was a totalitarian state—but so was the South. We had fought and died in a war between the same peoples, and the result was a standoff. Two dictatorships for the price of our blood, arms, legs, ears, eyes and penises. Precious lives surrendered involuntarily by my friends and colleagues, my brethren.

We forgot about that war quickly, Michael, and turned to other things. But the draft remained intact, ready to be geared up again when another set of old men decided it was time for the young to die. They found their cause, Michael, in Vietnam, only this time the cause was less clear, the honor less enobling. The trumpets were muted now, as we eased into the war between cousins and uncles. Why fight again? For the Free World? Of course. For mom and dad back home, to protect them against the communists? Sure. For the freedom of South Vietnam, so that they might live in peace? Under yet another dictator. And who the hell cared in 1965? No one. Michael, they took our kids again and demanded their lives. They stole that which belonged to the kids, that which could be given only by consent. For ten years we desecrated Vietnam and in the process we consumed our kids' lives much as a fireman uses up the water he sprays on a fire. But the cause was wrong, Michael, and even if it was right, the fifty-five thousand dead boys were not allowed to say no, I refuse to sacrifice my future. Three-hundred-thousand young bodies had no vote as the bullets and shrapnel seared and then punctured the skin and tore away kidneys, livers and scrotum. For what cause?

Michael, enough is enough. Gerald Ford, were you angry at the North Vietnamese for conquering the South? Did you tell us that our country was on the verge of disaster if the Cambodians grabbed a merchant ship on the high seas? If the North Koreans move in great numbers down past the thirty-eighth parallel and engulf South Korea, will the draft be reinstated in order to force the young to fight for you, Jimmy Carter? They will not, Mr. President. They will not be required, they will not be conscripted to make the ultimate sacrifice for you and the Generals. No more, Mr. Carter, we have ended the cycle of the young becoming cannon fodder for the politicians. Life is too noble to waste on emphemeral banterings that in the long run are unimportant.

Perhaps they will invoke that ultimate argument, Michael, in order to melt our resistance. Mr. Carter or some other President will say our country's very existence is at stake. They will dispute my Declaration of Independence by claiming that the enemy is invading our country, spilling over our shores, ravaging the land and our women. Could you stand by and refuse to be drafted to fight for your daughter's honor, Mr. Carter will ask. Michael, his argument is forceful and persuasive for many but not for me. If the cause is right we may volunteer for battle, but I do not relinquish my claim, that even under these grave circumstances, no President can force me to give up my life. My life is independent of local politics; my life is global. The principle I espouse is universal, cutting across the artificial boundaries of countries, language and culture. A life in America, translated to Vietnam is still a life, and is to be nurtured. Whomsoever possesses such a life is free to keep it under all circumstances.

Chapter 8
Neutralizing the Losses

In the cells, it may be metallic ions, enzymes and cellular materials together with oxygen which produce free radicals and hence initiate destructive oxidation processes. The free radical theory of aging deals primarily with the mechanism of oxygen utilization by the cells. Though degraded by oxygen, living systems also require oxygen in order to metabolize food for survival. So we have a mixed blessing. Some researchers are more concerned with the pathological damage caused by ozone which is a form of oxygen and suggest that ozone produces free radicals and is responsible for some pulmonary and non-pulmonary diseases we suffer in smog (which has a high ozone concentration). At sea level, the normal ozone content in air is on the order of 0.02 parts per million. But levels ten times this are not uncommon in Los Angeles where a 0.6 level has been recorded. Levels of 10 to 15 parts per million of ozone can kill small mammals in several hours. Thus ozone, beneficial to the extent that it screens our earth from excessive ultraviolet rays, may initiate damaging reactions in the body. As we produce more and more air pollution, we inexorably increase the ozone concentration in the air. Nature does exercise some moderating influence on the aberrations caused by free radicals and oxygen, and we observe that within the cells, there are naturally occurring antioxidants which neutralize some of the free radicals. The proponents of the free radical theory of aging contend that despite the presence of some naturally occurring antioxidants, there is nevertheless a continuous though small production of free radicals throughout our lifetimes, which causes damage and aging. Some antioxidants when fed to mice have apparently been a factor in extending their lifespan. Speculation on why these chemicals are effective in prolonging life range from their antioxidant properties as free radical scavengers, to their ability to help increase the formation of essential enzymes in the cells.

The discussion of oxygen and its toxicity and of antioxidants and their palliative effects leads quite naturally and relentlessly to vitamin E, which is supposed to possess antioxidant properties. Polyunsaturated fats are oxidized readily in the body; if this reaction is allowed to proceed at an unhindered rate, it can lead to serious diseased conditions. This potential is moderated by the presence of vitamin E, and some investigators have found a correlation between vitamin E needs for health and the fraction of the fats in the diet which is unsaturated. For example, too high a level of unsaturated fats in the diet can lead to sterility in rats, but this condition can be prevented by raising the ingestion level of vitamin E. In many studies, a direct connection was found between excess lipid oxidation (lipid peroxidation) and the degree of the vitamin E deficiency. We also know that the rate of oxidation of lipids in a cell is faster when the cells contain unsaturated fatty acids. Since vitamin E is an effective antioxidant, the logic of connecting lipid oxidation, unsaturated fats, free radicals, vitamin E, and aging is apparent. There is some disagreement as to whether vitamin E acts specifically as an antioxidant or only as one of the participants in the antioxidation process. And it may be that there are other chemicals which act similarly. Some materials have already been identified with long chemical names; but the toxicity and side effects of these free radical scavengers (antioxidants) are not fully established. Some of the data obtained using vitamin E substitutes are conflicting, suggesting to some researchers that traces of vitamin E are required for these substitutes to be effective. Another complicating factor in these studies is the realization that there are different forms of vitamin E. Thus one form of vitamin E (γ-tocopherol), abundantly present in corn oil, is effective in protecting red blood cell membranes from excessive oxidation damage, but it is only 10 percent as effective as another vitamin E form (α-tocopherol) in another application. The need for vitamin E in human nutrition is established but there is some disagreement on the amount required, which is not surprising since we know that there are a variety of species of vitamin E. The recommended daily dosage of vitamin E is: infants, 5 IU; children 1 to 10 years of age, 1 to 15 IU; adults, 20 to 30 IU. A study done in 1965 showed that our daily intake of vitamin E varied from 3 to 15 milligrams, with the average intake being 7.4 milligrams. If these data are correct, it would appear that some of us are not getting enough vitamin E into our systems. We know that the need for vitamin E depends directly on the amount of polyunsaturated fats in the diet and we also know that cooking tends to destroy the vitamin E content in foods. Some chronic disorders may be the result of a vitamin E deficiency and may be treated with large doses of vitamin E. (Large doses of this vitamin are not considered harmful.) Some researchers advocate a vitamin E intake of a few hundred IU's per day, with claims of beneficial effects in the treatment of diseases such as atherosclerosis, some heart conditions, diabetes, ulcers and muscular dystrophy. There is some preliminary evidence linking vitamin E to cholesterol levels in the blood.

The free radical theory of aging also connects with another theory of aging involving the production of age pigments such as lipfuscin. This colored material which seems to be inert and may be harmless metabolic debris, accumulates with age in tissue, especially in the heart and brain cells. It is believed that lipofuscin results from lipid and protein fragments which are generated by the peroxidation (excessive oxidation) of the cell membranes. Elevated pressures of oxygen produce cellular damage and death, apparently by increasing the rate of lipid peroxidation: Vitamin E protects mice from these hyperbaric oxygen disabilities. Vitamin E also protects mice against the lethality of ozone. Carcinogens induce chromosomal breakage in excess (10 to 20 percent) of the control group. Antioxidants reduce these chromosomal breakages by 30 to 65 percent. In experiments with human living cells which have the potential of producing about

50 doublings, when vitamin E was added to the cell broth, the cells continued to reproduce beyond 120 divisions. Food sources rich in vitamin E are egg yolk, fats, milk, peanuts and wheat germ oil. The average intake, which now may be up to 11 IU per day is thought to be less than the 20 to 30 IU's per day which is today our requirement for adults. Vitamin E influences the absorption of iron and affects the utilization of vitamin A. Vitamin E also improves the condition of children with hemolytic anemia and is effective in treating idiopathic nocturnal leg cramps. If the presence of free radical scavengers (antioxidants) affects the aging process, then by measuring the mercaptan levels, we should have a clue as to life expectancy. (Mercaptans are free radical scavengers.) Persons with high serum mercaptan levels could expect to live longer than those with lower values; those with low mecaptan levels should die faster. Vitamin C, vitamin A and niacin have properties much like the mercaptans and we find that old people (who die at a faster rate than young people) generally have low concentations of these chemicals. Older persons with low blood levels of vitamins A and C have a higher mortality rate than do their cohorts with higher blood levels of the two vitamins. Doesn't this suggest an experiment to you, whereby we assemble a cohort group of old people: one group gets enough vitamin C, niacin and vitamin A to maintain their serum concentrations at a "youthful" level. The other group is the control. Which group would live longer?

By feeding mice a diet of BHT (an antioxidant) it was possible to increase the age at which 50 percent of the mice were dead. In other experiments free radical inhibiters were added to the daily diet of mice. In going from 2 to 20 months, about 9 percent of the control group survived whereas 61 percent of those who were fed BHT survived. Other researchers were able to extend the lifespan of mice from 14.5 months to 18.3 months with 2-MEA. Attempts to extend life are related of course to an interest in nutrition. Vitamin E deficiencies, in addition to generating an accelerated free radical attack, may also lead to a reduction in cell membrane stability. Vitamin C deficiencies could also lead to a decreased cell membrane stability and might additionally yield shrunken collagen which will diminish tissue permeability, giving some cell impairment. Although there is ample controversy over vitamin C, it is clear that the body needs much more of it than simply for the prevention of scurvy. We now know that inflammation of the gums, loss of teeth, muscle pain, skin lesions and spontaneous hemorrhage result from defects in connective tissue which requires vitamin C for proper collagen synthesis. Ten milligrams a day may be sufficient to prevent scurvy but there are reasons for thinking that higher doses are needed for optimal health. Many factors influence the concentration of vitamin C in the blood and tissues. Blood levels of vitamin C are higher in women than men but are commonly reduced during pregnancy and lactation as well as by the use of oral contraceptives. Old age, cigarette smoking and the use of drugs, including aspirin also reduce the concentration of vitamin C in the blood. So do conditions of stress, trauma such as burns and surgery and infections including colds. It is also assumed that vitamin C is needed during wound healing because of the vitamin's known function in collagen synthesis. Thus high doses are often given to surgical patients. Guinea pigs when fed a normal diet but lacking in vitamin C developed high levels of cholesterol in the blood and liver. If extra cholesterol was added to the diet, it accumulated in various tissues including the aorta where it formed plaques similar to those seen in humans with atherosclerosis. Vitamin C fed with cholesterol to this group prevented the accumulation. A question arises, whether vitamin C could help prevent cancer caused by environmental carcinogens. The carcinogen 3-HoA which causes bladder cancer in mice is metabolically neutralized if vitamin C levels in the mice urine were kept high. Experimental animals can get cancer from consuming amines and nitrites which are preservatives in ham, bacon, frankfurters and smoked fish. Vitamin C fed to animals protects against tumor generation which might be caused by a diet of these food preservatives. With a body pool of vitamin C of about 1500 milligrams, three percent of the body pool was degraded per day. Thus, it was concluded that 45 milligrams per day was needed. Recommended daily allowances are not designed to cover increased needs resulting from severe stress, disease or trauma.

Disorders of the male prostate gland afflicting about one-third of the old men in our country apparently are prevented by eating sunflower or pumpkin seeds which correct the swelling and inflammation. These foods are rich in zinc. It has been found that ingestion of 50 to 100 milligrams of zinc can cause a shrinkage of swollen prostates in 14 of 19 patients in one study. (Areas of the world where a zinc deficiency is most common are Egypt and the Middle Eastern countries.) Oral supplementation of zinc accelerates wound healing. Surgical wounds produced in rats rendered zinc deficient have a lower tensile strength than others and healing is delayed. The zinc concentration in wound exudate is two to four times higher than in the associated plasma fluid. Abnormally low levels of zinc are found in patients with alcoholic cirrhosis and other liver disease, tuberculosis, myocardial infarcts, pulmonary infections, Down's Syndrome, cystic fibrosis as well as pregnant women and women taking oral contraceptives. Cases which respond positively to zinc therapy are leg ulcers, nutritional dwarfism and chronic ulcers. Oral administration of zinc sulfate for venus leg ulcers (200 milligrams, three times daily) gave no significant improvement in 30 days but after 40 days there was a remarkable healing of the ulcers. Our estimated dietary intake of zinc is 10 to 15 milligrams per day while the recommended dose is 15 milligrams per day. Zinc is found in high concentrations in seafood, animal meat, eggs, legumes and whole grain. It is thought that a zinc deficiency impairs RNA metabolism which may result in impaired synthesis of protein and nucleic acids. Dry sockets in dental patients with teeth removed improved by treatment with vitamin C, B-complexes and zinc sulfate. Oral intake of zinc can decrease claudication (a limp and lameness) and enhance tissue integrity in patients with atherosclerosis: though scheduled for surgery, they did not require an operation when treated extensively with zinc. Surgical patients who experience post-operative decreases of taste acuity were found to have low serum levels of zinc. Consuming zinc sulfate helped alleviate the problem. Administration of radioactively tagged zinc allowed researchers to pinpoint that zinc localizes in healing tissues and seems to improve the healing rate. With 200 milligrams of zinc sulfate administered three times a day there was an accelerated healing in 43 percent of the cases. As we get older there is a diminishing amount of zinc in our bodies; as we get older the healing process is less effective; zinc has been found to be useful in promoting wound healing and is used topically and even internally for this purpose in some hospitals; our daily intake of zinc, on the average, is marginal in meeting our daily requirements. Therefore, should we take zinc to help keep our daily intake above average, to attempt to maintain our blood serum levels high into old age and thus perhaps keep our healing process youthful?

Do the cells of an organ of the body regenerate if there is some loss of cells? One researcher implanted an inflated plastic pouch in place of a diseased bladder. In less than two months the first tissue layers of new bladder had grown. In three months a coating of smooth muscle tissue enclosed the inner layer, and soon the bladder regeneration was completed. The 3 inch by 4 inch plastic bag was then deflated and removed through the uretha. The nerve connections seemed good. In the liver, only one of 10,000 to 20,000 cells is in mitosis (dividing) at any time. If one of the lobes of the liver (about 70 percent of the liver) is removed, the remaining cells proliferate rapidly and reconstitute most of the original liver in a few days. Young rats can regenerate liver tissue more rapidly than adults. If there is some regeneration possible on the cellular level, doesn't this indicate that some aspects of the aging process are reversible? Young, middle-aged and old rats can apparently regenerate liver material equally well, but old rats do not produce as many cells containing nuclei as their younger brethren, suggesting that the new mass produced by old rats is not as functional as the new material generated by the younger ones. Experiments on the muscles of rabbits seem to indicate that some muscle regrowth is possible: the researchers ligated the blood supply of the gastrocnemius muscle of some rabbits and found that the muscle material was soon broken down and resorbed. Then the researchers restored the blood supply; after some further degeneration, there was a regrowth phase where new muscle was deposited. Soon nerve cells appeared and the muscle became functional—nearly as good as before. How is this possible? Why can't it be done in other animals and other parts of the body? Is there a need for a connective tissue frame upon which to build the new material? Some muscle tissue can be regenerated, but the process is not fully understood. Is this regeneration of tissue related to the observation that in the old there is greater time lag before a wound begins to heal than for the young? Salamanders can regenerate lost toes; sometimes they can even replace a foot. The cells beneath the scar tissue regain their embryonic state capabilities, begin to divide, and restore the original tissue patterns of the lost member. Soon the tissue has specialized as new bone, connective tissue, muscles and skin through which blood vessels extend themselves. Nerve cell regeneration is much slower. Earthworms regenerate as long as no serious injury is caused to the region between segments 4 and 30 where the vital organs are located. There are 180 segments in the body of an earthworm and when some segments are lost, they can be regenerated exactly (the same number are produced to replace those which were lost). Is this ability to replace lost portions of the body a sign of a higher order of life? Humans can't do what the salamander or the earthworm can do—yet.

In a human cell there are 46 chromosomes in the nucleus of each cell. Cell division takes about one day. A second division also takes about one day; subsequent divisions are slower. Nerve cells don't divide; skin cells do divide. Cancer cells that result from mitosis fail to align themselves smoothly against neighbors or to form neat mosaics. Instead they pile on top of one another When about 10,000 cells are clumped, then we see a tumor. It takes about 12 divisions starting from one cell to produce a noticeable lump. Cancer cells take about six days for each division; after 150 days there could be a mass 5/32 of an inch in size which is formed, the result of about 25 divisions. This is not the sort of regeneration we seek.

Chapter 9

Reflections In An Aging Eye

Yesterday, when I was young
The taste of life was sweet as rain upon my tongue
I tasted life as if it were a foolish game
The way the evening breeze may tease a gentle flame
The thousand dreams I dreamed
The splendid things I planned
I always built alas on weak and shifting sand
I lift my eyes and shine the naked light of day
And only now I see how the years ran away

Yesterday, when I was young
So many drinking songs were waiting to be sung
So many women with pleasure in store for me
And so much pain my dazzled eyes refused to see
I ran so fast that time and youth at last ran out
I never stopped to think what life was all about
And every conversation I can now recall
Concerns itself with me, me and nothing else at all

Yesterday, the moon was blue
And every crazy day brought something new to do
I used my magic age as if it were a wand
That never saw the waste and emptiness beyond
The game of love I played without angst and pride
And every flame I let too quickly, quickly die

The friends I made all seemed somehow to drift away
And only I am left on stage to end the play
There are so many songs in me that won't be sung
I feel the bitter taste of tears upon my tongue
The time has come for me to pay for
Yesterday, when I was young.

YESTERDAY WHEN I WAS YOUNG
by C. Aznavour and H. Kretzmer

Michael, I remember as a youngster, walking to school in bitterly cold weather, with hair originally wet but now frozen stiff, fingers cold, blood circulation seemingly nonexistent. My parents were aghast at my carelessness and indifference as I suffered from the exposure. I recall playing basketball in the schoolyard in the winter, after clearing the snow off the court. We removed coats, stripped to our undershirts and played for hours in the freezing cold; even I who was suffering from a cold and cough. Adrenalin pumping in my blood masked the cold symptoms while I played and then later stood around on the street corner talking and congealing. My parents quite naturally were horrified at this and then angry: what the hell was I trying to do? Kill myself? I coughed all night, a wracking, gut-shaking, intestine-cracking, hernia-inducing sequence of wrenches. But I recovered. I had no doubts that I would overcome the effects, that I would be as good as new.

Michael, I was always good at sports, being able to play the street games of punchball and stickball as well as baseball, basketball and football. Before the automobile stole our streets from us, we who spent so much time in the streets, on our block, were always able to round up a quorum and play at something. How easy it was in those days to run without gasping for breath, how glorious a feeling to swing a bat with all your might and not tear a muscle, to crash into each other thereby generating very painful cuts and bruises and then have them heal quickly without a trace. I could see so well, so clearly was the ball in my field of vision. If I saw it, there was always time to catch it or to hit it with quick, youthful reflexes. You, too, Michael are blessed with fine physical attributes and I envy you. Your strong, erect body will soon have the rippling muscles I once had, with the tight distensible flesh of youth. Your clear eyes can flash happiness and anger as mine did a long time ago. As a tennis player I could go for five sets of singles in the broiling sun, serving hard, attempting smashing overheads, covering the corners with grace and speed. But now I wear glasses to see, and my reflexes are considerably slowed. My hair is thinning and becoming coarse with a bare patch showing at the rear of my head, and some gray is growing. My skin has more wrinkles, I weigh the same as before but there is a certain slackness of skin around the middle. I get more tired more quickly than before and recover less rapidly.

But I am not depressed. Michael, I am armed with statistics which allay my fears. I am suffering nothing special, I am not a freak, I am running my life's course on schedule as all before me have done. I am just getting older. I cannot work as well at elevated temperatures as I used to, my tendency is to have more accidents. The strength in my muscles is diminished. Michael, my reaction time is down from its peak quickness and so is my back strength. Our cardiac function diminishes steadily into old age and so does breathing capacity. There is a loss in the ability of the lungs to let air through the lung membranes. As a general rule, we can say that there is a one percent loss in function for each year of life. Stomach acid secretions drop with age so it becomes more difficult to digest those spicy hot dogs and pickles, less blood is pumped through the kidneys, the metabolic rate drops as does one's nerve conduction velocity. How old are you? Michael, how old are your lungs? How old are your nerves? How old are your muscles?

Michael, as we get older an error once made is difficult to correct. We are losing speed and flexibility and reserves. I know this, Michael, and therefore understand more fully what is happening to me and that which transformed my father. I have become more accepting of my losses and considerably more tolerant of the plight of the old, as I hope you will be.

My father's father, my grandfather, your great grandpa, lived with us when I was growing up. Michael, we were crowded together in a three-room apartment, my father and mother, I and two brothers and our grandfather. My grandfather was the one to take me to the movies on the lower East Side of Manhattan when I was very young and he was still vigorous. My first recollection of films, indeed the first movie I went to was with my grandfather. Perhaps he didn't exercise such good judgement in the selections (there were no child psychologists available to advise us) for he and I went to my first film and saw a double feature: Frankenstein in one and Dracula in the other. Oh how I schemed that night. If Frankenstein came into our apartment, I would hide under the bed since he was too lumbering and dumb to look there for me. But if Dracula came, it was the closet for me—how else could you avoid a bat?

There were grand times with my grandpa, your great grandpa whom you never knew. But the later memories of him are not as pleasant, when he became retired from his everyday work which had vitalized his DNA and RNA. In his eighties, there was nothing seriously wrong with him—except he had nothing to do. He sat and sat and eventually began to generate the complaints of the old. He lost his sense of worth as did his son, my father, upon his own retirement. Michael, they say my grandfather became senile at home but I believe this condition was easily reversible if we could have challenged him. If we could have demonstrated how we needed him, that we were not going to allow him to sink into the pit of self-pity. He took to drumming on the kitchen table with his fingers as he sat and stared. It nearly drove me crazy, Michael, as I tried to do my homework. Who was this old man whom I no longer recognized? Where was my real grandfather, the man who carried me in his strong arms, who walked the Lower East Side with me, who led me on countless adventures?

Kids in New York develop early (perhaps prematurely) the knack for survival as they travel the underground railway called the subway. I was no exception, Michael, for in order to go to my high school, it was necessary to spend almost two hours each day on the subway. Ritualistically you gathered your money, enough for the round trip and walked to the subway entrance. In winter I froze waiting for the trains on platforms which seemed to concentrate the cold and dampness in the bone marrow. In late spring and early fall, the subway system seemed to act as a heat sink, drawing the warmth of the day and previous days into its bowels. While the fortunate bus and auto riders above ground enjoyed the spring and fall air, other human moles burrowed underground and sweated, in the heat which was magnified by the closely-packed, randomly-spaced human cargo. Michael, I hated those subway rides which were to continue through my college days. There is a rhythm of life underground, as you wait on the platform in expectation of the next train. If it comes quickly, you feel happy and rewarded, as if this day were to be your lucky one. What God is controlling my destiny? Whose diety has decided to send the train to me after only a thirty-second wait? Thank you, whoever you are. But if I must wait for longer periods, I curse the city and the Mayor and the trainman and all those other evil men joined in a conspiracy to ruin my day. There they are, drinking coffee and carousing, laughing as they watch me grimacing as I pace up and down the station. I look out over the tracks in the direction from which the train is to come. Then I glance down the tracks in the direction I hope to go. Is the light green? Good, nothing is wrong, but where is the train? And finally, Michael, my train came and I rushed to the spot on the platform that by experience, by a seemingly infinite number of trials, I knew would be the exact spot where the doors would be opened. Move in quickly, everyone, no delay or the door will clamp on your buttocks. Seats? Are there any empty ones? Walk quickly and determinedly to a seat and get down fast before some pregnant or very old lady blocks your path. I ignore everyone else. Regular subway riders don't give up their seats easily. We expect no advantages and give few favors. And there we sit in utter boredom, attempting to read a newspaper or a school book, glancing periodically at the people to measure their anatomy and also at the ads lining the walls. The rattling and shaking, the ear-splitting, high decibel, high pitched screeching dulls the senses, raises the blood pressure, irritates our nerve endings, wears out the eyes, mutes our hearing and grinds down our teeth. If ever the wear and tear theory of aging applied, it is in the subway. Crowded together unnaturally, with no privacy, no dignity, pushed here and there, manipulated by unseen, omnipotent forces, who can be at ease traveling in this chamber of horrors. And so we age, we wear out, we fall apart, the process catalyzed by the New York City subway which I used every day for four years of high school.

Michael, after the years on the block in grade school and high school, who was I? To what extent was I formed? How recognizable as the final product is a boy in high school? Do you know me, your father, any better now? My high school taught me mathematics (even some calculus), physics, chemistry, English and German, drafting and other mundane matters which soaked into my sponge-like innards. It was so easy to learn in those days, the mind seemed a magnet attracting knowledge. Facts and figures literally leapt into my brain, captured and reorganized for later regurgitation on examinations. Grade school had also seemed simple, even easier than high school. Is this impression accurate, was my brain at the top of its form? The brain is probably at its peak performance during the teens, having grown in size steadily, achieving about ninety percent of its final weight by age four and its final maximum mass by about ten years of age.

Actually, Michael, I cannot accurately recall very much about my high school days except going and coming, and spending the rest of the time back on the block. There were good teachers and bad ones, old and young, easy and strict, but one thing I do remember vividly: there were no girls in my high school. How awful, I know now, that I was deprived of the daily association, the daily socialization so important in learning. Not just book learning, Michael, but that learning which is preparation for life, allowing humans to live and love in society. We were a gang of rowdies at times, resembling acned college fraternity "men" in the worst pejorative sense. Who was the organizer of this dreadful style of educational life and learning? What masochist, what pervert, what bitter spinster or uptight male prude declared my high school off limits to girls. So Michael, I learned from books but missed a lot of other things which make me, even today, feel deprived. Thus did my years quickly and unknowingly slip by, Michael. Twenty to thirty percent of my life was already spent and I was learning from books but living little, oblivious of the world beyond my ethnic block, unaware of the outside world, unable to savor the other dimensions of education which develop outside the classroom.

I would have changed much if I could, Michael, to alter the routine into which I was locked in those days. You shall not be as deprived as I was, Michael. I will carry you beyond the classroom, you shall have the opportunity to transcend elementary book learning. I shall challenge your mind and spirit, you shall meet situations which cause you to connect seemingly uncoordinated facts and events, your brain shall swell with the exercise. I shall be present, Michael, my son. My essence will impinge on your being. We shall play and work together and separately, sometimes side by side. We shall not waste time and life, you shall find time to play and love. You shall know life, you will learn to love life, your vitality shall not be wasted. I shall read to you and you shall read to me. We will talk, we shall communicate one-on-one, as father and son and as two human beings. I shall respect you as a person and as my son. I shall grant you all the basic human rights and I pray you will reciprocate. Michael, my child, my son, I will this to you and me.

It is the invariant sequence of life, that we are born, grow to maturity and then decline at an ever increasing rate of deterioration. Thus, Michael, did I arrive at college in New York City, eighteen years of age, already into the early-mature phase of life and still appallingly inexperienced. Who was I? Did I understand the forces at work which were molding my psyche? There are those who say that we are born fully formed and spend our lives developing the latency inherited. I believe this, to an extent, Michael. I see it in you very clearly and in retrospect I suppose for me it was a matter of finding the instrumentality.

Thus I began the by now very familiar subway trek, this time to college. But now there was a difference. Michael, I was prepared to accept a different culture, I was ready to measure what I knew against new information presented to me. My brain, my social mores, my entire fabric were fertile and awaiting some sort of intercourse. And so I began the metamorphosis, emerging a few years later from the ethnic, block-oriented local yokel form to the more reasonable approximation of my final self. During this intermediate stage there was a heady new freedom but also a deep sense of loneliness and loss. The old friends on the block were now vestigial and soon we drifted apart. My parents who provided the early support, the safety which I required, understood that irresistable forces were at work. They instinctively sensed the esoteric, unverbalized pressures focused here and that they must step back. Michael, it was a time of great tensions for me and them. That adjustment was made more difficult for me, as I encountered twenty-five hours of class work each week and tremendous quantities of home work assigned by each professor who assumed his subject was the only one which was important. And then there were the subway rides which sapped your vitality on each end of the day. I carried my lunches from home and ate my suppers in a nearby cafeteria in order to keep up with the routine. I studied in the college library at night.

It was a high price to pay, Michael, acquiring an education under these adverse conditions while suffering the evolutionary pangs. Michael, the human organism is remarkably resilient and powerful, particularly in the early-mature stage of development. But the wear and tear took its toll as my eyes gave out and physical and mental exhaustion encroached. My grades were not great, but I had made the quantum leap beyond the old confines. I could now think and write as a universalist, seeing the world as an interconnected network with feedback mechanisms clearly at work. We depended on each other, Michael, the whole world did, and what we did here affected them there. Thus was born within me—or finally synthesized—a sensitivity to humaneness and human dignity and a desire to work on important concerns of mankind. My thoughts were appropriately primitive, still not polished, but nevertheless recognizable and would require another twenty years to become coherent. But they were there, I knew it, and awaited the opportunity.

What was lost during this process, Michael? I lost my block which was my security, my homeland. The old buddies became distant, casual acquaintances to be greeted with embarrassed, empty banter. Michael, I lost my family, my parents especially, as I struggled to find myself. My parents, already long into the late-mature phase of life were fully formed and declining. They were them, and I was me and there was a difference. Nothing unique was happening here, Michael, it has been seen before. But I must impress this upon you, so that when it happens to us, you will understand. Michael, there is a happy ending here, as I shall tell you later. I found my parents again after a period of years during which I too became fully formed. I finally understood more about the aging process as applied to the human condition, and in particular to me and my parents. So while they were suffering the losses of old age, I was developing, maturing and discovering. Then, at the magic moment, parents and child merged again after a long separation. Luckily it was not too late.

# Chapter 10
Mutations

There are other categories of aging, such as the somatic mutation theory of aging which states that (1) spontaneous mutations of cells, propagated by cell divisions, cause the formation of inferior cells and (2) mutated cells form more often in old individuals. Since most mutations are harmful, the living system, with age, becomes less efficient and eventually is unable to survive. Those who promote the mutation theory say that the mutated cells stimulate immunologic reactions within the organism which eventually destroy or weaken the host functions and we die. Somatic mutationists proclaim further their belief that spontaneous mutations build up in both dividing and non-dividing cells. Non-dividing cells such as aging red blood cells have increasing numbers of abnormal cohorts. Discussion of mutations in cells leads naturally to DNA which constitutes the chromosomes of the nucleus. A single DNA molecule is responsible for each function in the cell, such as replication during cell division (through RNA messenger units which the DNA produces). RNA diffuses out into the cell cytoplasm where it synthesizes a particular enzyme. Mutagenic agents are thought to damage the DNA and eventually kill or alter the cell. The most difficult task for a cell is the division process, since the cell needs all of its DNA for this operation. Irradiated cells appear normal until cell division occurs when they may die or give bizarre daughter cells.

In living and dying, chemicals within the cells are synthesized, degraded and rejected or resorbed. Some materials, like DNA, once synthesized do age but are not readily degraded. On the other hand, RNA apparently can disappear, having a half-life of one hour or less. More RNA must be continuously generated. Somehow, the enzymes which degrade or break down age-altered molecules are able to recognize the difference between young and old. They selectively degrade the old, which are replaced by a young, newly synthesized population. In the body, some cells undergo regular divisions (skin) or rarely divide (liver) or never divide (brain). It is thought that mutations in cells which undergo regular divisions cause little permanent damage to the organ involved, since the mutated cells will die or lose out in the competition with other cells. Some researchers think that organs which have non-dividing cells should ultimately be responsible for the aging process and senescence. They cite the example of blood-forming organs (with dividing cells) which function far into old age whereas muscles (non-dividing cells) show the first signs of aging. However, non-dividing cells can apparently function nearly normally for long periods with damaged chromosomes—using up the previously formed, normal RNA of the cytoplasm. Mammalian dividing cells can frequently continue three to five divisions after a moderate dose of radiation before the daughter cells die or become bizarre; mammalian non-dividing cells (red blood cells) function normally for a long time without a nucleus. The somatic mutationists proclaim that the genetic structure of the cells, in the chromosomes, carry the function and instructions; when the chromosomes are damaged, there could be a synthesis of wrong proteins. The errors will be propagated by the daughter cells. The mutations will accumulate until a significant portion of the organism is "aged" and eventually dies. X-rays which cause mutations are known to shorten life expectancy in proportion to the dosage. The victim assumes the characteristics of a naturally aged person so one concludes that there is an aging destructiveness to radiation. But radiation results are not intrinsically germane to the somatic mutation hypothesis, since the radiation is an external stress imposed and thus any support these data provide is beneficial only by inference. There is evidence for support of the idea that mutations occur more frequently in short-lived animals than in long-lived ones and that this is the "reason" for differences in lifespan. But we haven't dealt with the question,—the more significant aspect of our search for the truth—of why the mutations occur. There is no answer to this question from the somatic mutationists. Not everyone agrees that the somatic mutation theory is the most probable or the only theory which can explain the process of aging. The dissenters say that too many other factors are known to be involved. Even in cancers induced by radiation, some believe that it is not the mutated cells which finally form the cancer. They cite the evidence that we can increase the incidence of mutations in an organism, yet tumor frequency is not proportional to the number of mutations. And the diminishment of life expectancy does not keep pace either. Also, there is some time lag between the production of mutations and the tumors which are generated, which seems unreasonable to some researchers, particularly unreasonable when in some cases this latent period is 40 years. We also have identified "precancerous tissue" which beclouds the logical connection between mutations, aging and cancer. There may be thousands of cells in a tissue sample, and skeptics find it difficult to allow that a cancerous mutation has occurred simultaneously in all of these cells. Further, it has been found that some strains of mice which die of leukemia at about 10 months of age do not develop chromosome aberrations in their liver cells any faster than nonleukemic strains. So there are plenty of doubters for every proponent of the somatic mutation theory of aging. After x-radiation, the number of chromosome aberrations returns to the control level of the untreated animals, so that in some cases, while the increased death rate is being felt, the chromosome aberration count is normal. This seems to point to some inconsistency in the logic employed by the somatic mutationists.

Mutation in the genes may lead to a mutated cell which misidentifies itself to its cellular neighbors, evoking reprisals against the mutation—and perhaps against its normal neighbors. In relating aging to immune reactions, some investigators suggest that we have, due to mutations, a breakdown in the mechanism which normally prevents lymphocytes from producing antibodies antagonistic towards its own body material. With age, the mutated lymphocytes may produce antibodies which attack the host organism. This line of reasoning places the mutational process in the antibody producing cells rather than in the tissue cells and avoids the illogic of somatic mutation theory which says that aging is caused by a cell by cell mutation procedure—a relatively slow process. Radiation may raise the somatic mutation rate, but that alone would not seem able to account for the aging process. Thus we conclude that something else is at work in aging, in addition to somatic mutation: a suspicion that antibodies may be involved. An error in the antibody producer needs only one mutation followed by rapid clonal multiplication and we have the possibilities of the extensive, progressive damage we recognize as old age.

Chapter 11
Work

There is a ubiquitous malevolence contaminating our country these days, destroying the best of minds, the most honest of souls, the strongest of resolve, the most empathetic of spirits. It is called work. Why do we work? Most of us work for a living, which means working for survival and isn't that a horrible thought. You must spend eight hours a day, plus time in transit to and from the job, in order to collect money to pay for the privilege of living. You work in order to live. So the man on the assembly line tightens the same nut on the same bolt which periodically reappears, all replicas of the original, all hinged on indistinguishably alike cars moving always at the same speed down the assembly line. This human being slaves at his job, deferring his real life until the work day is completed. Do not think, mister, just keep doing your thing exactly the same way each time. Not too tight, not too loose, just right. Mister, do you ever worry about the loss of brain cells you suffer as you age on the assembly line? Do you think about your loss of strength and coordination? About the hair that is greying and that skin which is thinning and becoming wrinkly? You must worry about your sex life and your wife's and know that she and you will suffer a menopause which will stress your relationship. Keep twisting the nut, old man, where did your youth go? Were you young when you started this morning?

There are so many jobs in our society similar to the assembly line bore. Why must it be so? If we could understand that jobs use our time and time is life and life is finite, perhaps we would more often equate work and life and therefore waste neither. I have worked for a living, when I graduated from college as an engineer. How exciting it was, to be a young man, the chosen one among older, wiser heads, ready to move up in life, up the chain of command, as I acquired experience and knowledge. And the pay was very good. But, after the euphoria subsided, after the initial, introductory phase was over, I settled into a dull, repetitious, non-learning situation, unable to grow, far removed from the seat of power, with no voice in the decisions which affected my life and that of the company. It wasn't a situation exactly analogous to the dead-end condition of the assembly line workers but if you stripped away the fancy title and the relatively high wages, our jobs were not so dissimilar. And as my time was being wasted on unimportant matters, my life was draining away in vain. So, we parted, my company and me, one year after I graduated from a demanding college experience which had left me already mentally and physically exhausted.

Why must jobs be so circumspectly drawn, so practical, so much in favor of the company? Why doesn't some humanistically oriented tax-free foundation study the jobs in America and list the dead-end, dehumanizing ones. Warn everyone, educate us all. It is not that the assembly line job is so terrible in itself, for in the short run we could do it, given the need. But the prospect of doing it forever, day in and day out until we die (or get old enough to retire), with no possibility of advancement, that is the hangup. That is the crime of the assembly line. It is important for the human organism to think, to hope, to aspire and to love every day. Nothing of importance should be deferred for too long, for later may be too late as our lives run their course. Why can't we humanize our jobs by allowing time off during the day, once a week or perhaps more often, for the working stiff to pursue the things he chooses for himself, for his own purpose. Why not allow him to study painting or algebra or sports? Why can't he study metallurgy to help him on the job and other subjects which will permit and facilitate advancement to more inspiring work? Why shouldn't he have time off to plan for mid-career corrections, so that he may change directions, so that the assembly line operator might train for an accounting job? Why not plan for retirement, using the free time to learn of the dangers and opportunities of retirement? We know that assembly line operators will be as unprepared for retirement and as unable to cope with it as my father and his father were. There must be a period of adjustment and we know it can't come afterwards. So let them do it now, while they are still working, while still reasonably healthy, while able to see retirement in abstract terms. Afterwards there seems to be little we can do to alter the pattern ingrained into the nervous system.

You may have to work for survival. I hope not. I pray you will be fortunate and be able to work at life, to find something to do which will instill pride, which has some redeeming value and be beneficial for you and your cohabitants of this earth. It is the ennobling toil which gives you, as an individual, a justification for existing. It becomes an enhancer of the human spirit and the life process rather than a demeaner of it—as the assembly line job is now. I think I have found such a way of life, such a job, and am very happy. I hope you are as fortunate.

Chapter 12

Collagen: Stiff and Stiffer

We know that the amount of water in our bodies diminishes with age, while concomitantly the cells shrink. Thus do we, you and I and everyone else, become diminished. The water in our bones is believed to be replaced by collagen, which is the fibrous constituent of bone, cartilage and connective tissue. We get stiffer with age, which is not news for those who try to stay athletic and graceful in their later years. And it has to do with our connective tissue, which in the aged is not as distensible as it was earlier. This connective tissue binds and supports other things in the body, such as the tendons, ligaments, skin, blood vessels, bone, teeth, the lining of the gastrointestinal tract, and the lungs. Connective tissue is composed of collagen, elastin and other proteins. As we age, this connective tissue is less extensible; a general feeling of rigidity creeps into our bones. Collagen which makes up about one-third of the total body protein, is present in and around blood vessels and the heart. The passage of material into and out of blood vessel walls is through collagen, and so it is apparent that the condition (permeability) of the collagen is critical for proper bodily functions. If our collagen becomes stiff and excessively cross-linked, this will limit flexibility, the heart will not be able to constrict as well as it might, thus putting a strain on it. Large arteries become stiffened also. There is a diminished passage of gases, nutrients, metabolites, antibodies, and toxins through the vessels. Hypertension can result, hypoxia (lack of oxygen) can occur in the cells —possibly causing them to become neoplastic—and cancer may result. Aged connective tissue is more easily invaded by tumors. But there are puzzling data which give rise to uncomfortable doubts about the relationship between collagen and tumors. It is known that the incidence of tumors does not increase steadily with age but seems to appear overwhelmingly only at advanced age. If the collagen theories are reasonable, tumors should appear at a steady rate from birth to death. Perhaps they do, but then the body is somehow able to neutralize them when we are young. Collagen is synthesized as soluble molecules that aggregate to form insoluble collagen fibrils. With age, we get more and more insoluble collagen fibrils.

Researchers who study the aging process have always noted the similarities between aged human skin and tanned leather. Chemical tanning of leather is actually a cross-linking of cells which become bound to their neighbors—suggesting an analogy between this occurrence and that which occurs to the aging protein of the skin. Extending this cross-linking concept uniformly for all organs of the body, one can speculate on the possibility of serious, fatal harm being done to living systems as a result of cross-linking of large molecules in the body. Early in this century it was demonstrated that for large molecules, one cross-linkage for every 30,000 components is enough to drastically change the solubility and behavior of the molecule.

Within the living cell, DNA has a particular steric configuration; should some disruptive agent appear, two or more DNA molecules may be tied together by cross-linking some of their components, seriously disturbing the effectiveness of the DNA. Many changes in function will result, particularly serious is the generation of missynthesized materials which cannot be acted upon normally by the body enzymes. Thus these "foreign" bodies may accumulate, crowding out other constituents, causing a decline in cell function. There could be molecular havoc produced by cross-linking, with the normal, precise arrangements of proteins and enzymes in the cells and membranes badly disrupted and their biological activities stymied. Collagen and elastin seem to manifest the effects of cross-linking most dramatically between ages 30 and 50 years in humans, caused by a "tanning" or formaldehyde-like chemical reaction. Proponents of cross-linking say that aging is caused by increasing cross-linkages of protein and nucleic acid molecules, leading to progressive deterioration of chemical performance and eventual death of the organism. Cross-linking can also take place between large molecules such as DNA and smaller, "cross-linker types", capable of reacting with two different large molecules and thereby forming a bridge between the large ones. This reduces the mobility of the linked molecules and leads to the formation of aggregates which have new diffusion properties as well as altered permeability and other essential characteristics. The damage to DNA is probably that of a cross-linking of two helices, making it impossible for one of the helices to act as a template in repairing the other. The principal effect of radiation is thought to be a cross-linking one; the other result of irradiation is a chain splitting effect, but it is thought now that the fragments which are produced from the fission are usually small enough to be excretable. Thus we see that cross-linking and radiation concepts are intermingled. Perhaps the various theories of aging, though presented as separate entities, are in actuality all part of an overall scheme of aging which is not yet developed.

Unsaturated fats, when oxidized, form some aldehydes and peroxides which are cross-linkers. With all of these materials present in the cells in relative abundance, it is frequently asked why the aging process in humans does not proceed rapidly to its conclusion in a matter of months rather than decades. The answer seems to be that there is a steady breakdown of mildly cross-linked protein molecules into simpler constituents and a resynthesis of these components into viable, non-cross-linked materials. Hence, there is a rapid turnover of protein, a reasonable balance of errors is struck, and the aging process then proceeds at a more moderate pace.

The character of the cross-linked material apparently varies from organ to organ, depending on the animal species, nutritional factors, and other more indefinite things. With age, humans seem to concentrate metallic materials in arteries; analysis of the human aorta shows evidence of metallic oxides in the cross-linked tissue. Other locations show no metal concentrations. With overfeeding, it is suspected that body metabolism cannot readily oxidize the foods to the usual water and carbon dioxide, but also forms intermediate products of metabolism. Some of these intermediates are powerful cross-linkers and could accelerate the aging process. This is consistent with experimental evidence which indicates that obese or very well nourished persons have shorter lifespans than underfed, healthy individuals. The cross-linking (collagen) believers propose that their theory of aging allows for the progressive reduction with age of the ability of hormones, enzymes and other essential materials to diffuse into and out of their active sites. Thus the life process slows down say the cross-linkers. Transmission speeds of nerve impulses are down, among other things, and the living, dynamic system becomes progressively sluggish. Cross-linking agents are so varied that avoidance of the agents in the diet or environment is impossible. If the effect of overeating is to produce a larger than normal concentration of deleterious cross-linking agents, then it is argued that many small meals would be preferable to a few large ones. (It has been shown that intermittent fasting periods are beneficial for maximum lifespan attainment.) Ingesting sufficient vitamin E and other antioxidants would be expected to be effective in neutralizing those cross-linkers which result from the oxidative process in the body (such as aldehydes and peroxides from unsaturated fatty acids). Cross-linkers in the cell membranes could be minimized by treatment with tocopherols (vitamin E) and other antioxidants of this genre. Researchers of the cross-linking persuasion also promote the use of dietary means for supplying a surplus of scavengers for the cross-linked molecules. Now if the scavengers do their jobs, and if the breakdown products are easily excretable from the body, then the progressive effect of cross-linking and aging can be moderated. The cross-link theorists also suspect that bad things come from metals such as copper, cadmium, lead, aluminum and silicon, which are known to increase in concentration with age and accumulate in "aged" organs. If these metals could be removed from the body by use of chelating agents, would cross-links be reduced and hence would the aging process also decline? Some researchers have shown that the lifespan of sea urchin spermatoza are multiplied several times if these metals are removed by chelating agents. Some think this procedure could be successful in rejuvenating the circulatory system in humans. It is suggested that it might be beneficial in the aged to use zinc salts to displace cadmium.

What we are looking for is a way of reversing the aging process, whereby we would break down the excessively cross-linked materials in the cells and make the cellular space available for other "normal" anabolic processes which could rejuvenate the cells. This can apparently be done for collagen in the uterus of rats, where cross-linked collagen can be made to be resorbed. If it is possible for one type of protein, can we do it for other proteins? We ought to seek these wondrous cross-link breakers from enzymes of soil bacteria, led in this direction apparently by the knowledge that some soil bacteria do break down fossil protein and thus there must be some enzymes present which make this possible. One of the enzymes might be our magic bullet. If the enzyme also attacked other proteins, this wouldn't be too objectionable as long as the normal anabolic processes of the body replaced the healthy protein which was removed. There is some evidence that proteolytic enzymes (which break down proteins into fragments) can actually reach the cells of the liver and kidney when given orally. Does this suggest an experimental approach? Some investigators say that old cross-linked collagen in wounds can be broken down. So the search goes on for an effective proteinase (protein enzyme) which will have an affinity for cross-linked material. We search for that magic bullet which can dissolve the old, stiffened, cross-linked collagen and allow it to be replaced by the young, more porous stuff. Thus would we have the regeneration we have sought for as long as we have known death? As we get stiffer with age by the cross-linking of our collagen we lose our grace and agility. It is natural and relentless, these changes, and we must live with the fact. Perhaps we can really slow the process by eating moderately with more numerous, smaller meals. Perhaps we can determine the effects of certain metallic elements on the rate of aging and substitute another for the ill-doer. We can invoke these minimal measures; certainly the dietary approach is easily done. If you accept the cross-linking ideas, along with the wear and tear theory, we should promote a calmer, less frenetic way of life, with the avoidance of excesses which insult our bodies and minds.

Chapter 13

Lost Horizons

Ah, look at all the lonely people

Eleanor Rigby, picks up the rice in the church where a wedding has been
Father McKenzie, writing the words of a sermon that no one will hear
Look at him working, nobody came

Eleanor Rigby died in the church and was buried along with her name
Lives in a dream
Waits at the window no one comes near
Wearing a face that she keeps in a jar by the door
Darning his socks in the night when there's nobody there
Wiping the dirt from his hands as he walks from the grave
Who is it for? What does he care? No one is saved

All the lonely people
Where do they all come from?
All the lonely people
Where do they belong
      Eleanor Rigby by John Lennon and Paul McCartney

    Our brains, like our muscles, require exercise and steady use in order to maintain optimal tone and function. I discovered this for myself when after being discharged from the army I enlisted in the graduate school at the University of Tennessee. It had been about three years since the undergraduate days in New York had exhausted me with the tension and overly long hours associated with attaining a very modest first college degree. It wasn't an easy transition, after three years, for I now found it difficult to think again, or, perhaps to put it more accurately, I found it difficult to begin to think. There were days and nights when by sheer concentration I forced my brain to open up new avenues for thought and analysis, stretching the blood vessels to give me more blood and oxygen. I could feel my mind expanding.

I had the good fortune to rent a room in the home of an old, widowed lady, a seventy-year-old possessing faulty eyesight, wrinkled skin, white hair, stooped and unsteady on her feet, with the creaky, weak voice of the old. But she was a swinger inside, she still worked, drove a car reasonably well, wrote poetry, aspired to a better life, yearned to be alive and loved her children and grandchildren. For this gentle old lady in Tennessee, in whose house I lived for three years, being needed, having something useful to do, having considerable self-esteem, writing and thinking about the world and enjoying the esthetics of living added up to a vital life force which energized her. She knew of death and was aware that she might die momentarily. But there was a higher calling and there were things to do and feel before that time came. And she did live, for a full ten more years until she became unable to work and drive. Then, the familiar, heartbreaking sequence of episodes began which leads to the usual end. She was convinced by relatives to give up her house, her homestead, her bedrock, her link with her self-esteem, because her children felt she could no longer care for herself. What a common mistake, to take from her what she needed so desperately: a sense of ownership, a link with her responsible past, something to work for. Instead she became dependent, a dependent child. What to do? Where to go? They invited her to come to the city where some of her children lived, to join a retirement home. I visited her there often and when we met, she displayed the brave face of the fighter but I sensed she was defeated. Who could she talk with, she asked. Most everyone there sat and vegetated and she wished to think. She worked at arts and crafts in a vacuum for there was no genuine appreciation of what she did. She read her poetry to an uninterested audience. There was no hope, no possibility of escape and soon the degenerative forces, awaiting the first signs of weakness, began to encroach upon her mentality. This led to diminished physical capability which in turn affected her mental functioning which reduced further her health. So the cycle continued and accelerated and shortly thereafter, too soon after entering this institution, this nice old lady died, looking just like all the other faceless, formless residents.

Why do we incarcerate our aged? Why do we disengage them from us, removing them from our sight? Is it that we fear them, seeing them as a portent of our own future? Why do we refuse to allow the young and the old to mingle? Is it for the sake of the old or is it that we cannot face our responsibilities to the past? Is it obdurateness, insensitivity, ignorance and fear? Why won't we be saddled by the cost and inconvenience of finding a way to allow the elderly to continue to live amongst us. We can't afford it we say and then spend our treasure in other, less humane ways. It interferes with our way of life, they slow us down as we search for pleasure and our need to earn a living. It is unpleasant to look at an old person so we segregate them in isolated institutions. Do we owe them anything? What do we owe that woman who was a poet, a mother, a grandmother and now is old? Does she have anything meaningful to say to us, to our children?

We now know that the old are capable of doing much more than we have previously attributed to them. Their systems function not as well as ours, but they work reasonably well. Given enough time the old can contribute, if not extended beyond their vital capacity. They can respond to stresses and work at a productive pace. So why do we send them to the garbage heap? We probably fear death; we probably fear the face of death which is mirrored in their faces. But there is nothing to fear. Living and dying are natural occurrences. It is only a matter of dignity. Shall we be born, live and die in dignity? Shall we agree that death is to be a peaceful event, not to be caused by war or as a result of someone's whim, but is to be allowed to happen at the pleasure of the recipient, the owner of that life? Can we agree that we accumulate dignity credits in life, that the elderly are entitled to spend these credits for care and respect where and when they choose and we the youngsters must honor their wishes. Where they live is important, but this does not mean institutional living for all the elderly as now is usually commanded, but if they wish, housing with and amongst their younger friends and relatives. Honor thy father and thy mother but give them more than that. They need contacts with all of us. We can benefit from such experiences. Will you do this for me?

Chapter 14
Nutrition Against Aging

Nutritional considerations are now a legitimate subject for discussion when we treat elderly patients. And for youngsters also (a derivative of vitamin A, 13-cis-retinoic acid, shows promise in the treatment of acne). Vitamin A in massive doses seems to condition smokers to be less apt to get lung cancer.[1] Vitamin C increases the absorption of iron from the intestines, a fact of importance to women. Vitamin D promotes the absorption of calcium and phosphorous into bone from the intestine; elderly women who are most prone to suffer from osteoporosis should take note of this. The major fat soluble vitamins are A, D, E and K; the major water soluble vitamins are thiamine (B_1), niacin (nicotinic acid), riboflavin (B_2), pyridoxine (B_6), pantothenic acid, folic acid, vitamin B_{12}, biotin and vitamin C. Dietary sources and effects of a deficiency in these vitamins are shown below.

Vitamin	Food	Traditional Symptoms of a Deficiency
A	fish, liver, eggs, butter, cheese, milk, green vegetables, carrots	night blindness, eye inflammation
D	fish, liver, butter, salmon	rickets, osteomylacia, hypoparathyroidism
E	vegetable oils, margarine, green leafy vegetables, grains, fish, eggs, meats	anemia
K	spinach, green leafy vegetables, tomatoes, vegetable oils	increased clotting times, bleeding under the skin

---

1. Sanders, H.J., Nutritional health, Chemical & Engineering News, March 26, 1979, 27-46

Vitamin	Food	Traditional Symptoms of Deficiency
Thiamine (B_1)	cereal, grains, nuts, milk, beef	beriberi
Niacin (nicotinic acid)	meat, liver, fish, eggs, peanuts	pellegra
Riboflavin (B_2)	milk, meat, liver, green vegetables, whole wheat, fish, eggs	dermatitis, anemia
Pyridoxine (B_6)	eggs, meat, peas, milk	dermatitis, convulsions in infants, infection
Pantothenic Acid	liver, beef, milk, eggs, peas	depression, mental confusion
Folic Acid	liver, green leafy vegetables, wheat, bran	anemia, gastrointestinal disorders
B_{12}	meat, fish, eggs, milk	anemia, retarded growth
Biotin	liver, peanuts, eggs, milk	dermatitis
C	citris fruits, tomatoes	scurvy

Aside from this traditional nutritional information, new claims have arisen, more esoteric benefits to be accrued: large doses of niacin may be useful in the treatment of schizophrenia; iron is useful in assisting in the generation of hemoglobin; iodine aids thyroid function; chromium is an activator of insulin production; cobalt helps in the synthesis of vitamin B_{12}. Zinc which is a constituent of more than 90 enzymes in our bodies is needed in insulin production, growth, cell division, pituitary, adrenal gland, pancreas and gonad function. A zinc deficiency can lead to depressed taste acuity, poor wound healing, loss of a sense of smell and a diminished immune response. Boys in Egypt who were deficient in zinc showed retarded growth, delayed sexual development and enlarged livers. Their zinc deficiency was found to be caused partly by their large consumption of bread containing high concentrations of dietary fiber which inhibits the absorption of zinc from the intestine. Some preschool children in Denver in 1972 who ate very little meat were found to be zinc deficient and growth retarded. Copper is the ever present component of the enzymes of the body involved with the utilization of oxygen. With a copper deficiency we tend to lose our hair pigment (copper helps form tyrosine which becomes the coloring material melanin), suffer from anemia and impaired bone formation.

Trace Element	Dietary Source	Functions in Humans and Others
iron	meat, liver, fish, poultry, beans, peas, raisins, prunes	in blood hemoglobin and some enzymes
iodine	iodized salt, shellfish	needed to synthesize thyroxine and triiodothyronine of the thyroid, prevents goiter
zinc	meat, liver, eggs, shellfish	in at least 90 enzymes and insulin
copper	nuts, liver, shellfish	in some enzymes, helps absorb iron
manganese	nuts, fruits, vegetables, whole-grain cereals	in some enzymes, bone
cobalt	meat, dairy products	part of vitamin B12
selenium	meat, seafood	in enzymes, helps fat metabolism
chromium	meat, beer, unrefined wheat flour	in glucose metabolism

A manganese deficiency can lead to bone abnormalities, defective egg shells in chickens, weight loss, slow growth of hair and nails and a reddening of the hair. Without adequate selenium in the body, we tend to suffer liver and kidney ailments and kwashiorkor. Fiber in the diet is recognized as essential, especially for older persons whose teeth and gums are sometimes unable to handle bulky, chewy fiber-containing foods. Low fiber diets are associated with colon cancer, diverticulitis and gall stones. We can get fiber from wheat and grains in general, fruits and vegetables. The beneficial effect of high fiber diets seems to be an increased excretion of cholesterol into the bloodstream which lowers cholesterol in the rest of the body. Consider this curious observation: rats fed corn as the only source of protein were found to have an unusually high sensitivity to pain, particularly electric shock. Corn contains tryptophan, a precursor to serotonin, a neurotransmitter. Can we connect this logical chain? Does serotonin in the brain have anything to do with responsiveness to pain in particular and stimuli in general?

The estimated intake of ascorbic acid (vitamin C) is a little higher than the recommended value.[1] Elderly patients in a long-term care facility tended to have vitamin C levels in their bodies in proportion to their ages: older means less. This suggests that for the elderly, vitamin C supplements ought to be regularly prescribed with sufficient testing to confirm maximally high tissue levels. Can we not do the same for vitamin E? Rats fed diets rich in vitamin E showed less lipofuscin in the brain. And what is the connection between this old age pigment and senility and changes in brain function in general? We believe magnesium is important in the diet since calcium absorption in bone is difficult without it.[2] A one percent increase in magnesium in the diet doubles bone density. Some dentists say magnesium is the key to our resistance to tooth decay. The combination of zinc and magnesium synergistically accelerates the healing of inflammations. Vitamins C and E are also effective. Cohen[3] summarized the improved longevity results obtained by McCay and others in the classic underfeeding experiments and adds another parameter: the protein level. He suggests, all things being equal, less protein is better. Garlic and onions seem to lower our chances of suffering thrombosis strokes (blood clots in our blood vessels)[4] by inhibiting blood platelet aggregation (makes them less "sticky"). Garlic and onions contain sulfur components which interfere with the synthesis of thromboxine, one of the steps in platelet aggregation. In a group of centenarians appearing before a congressional committee in Washington, all admitted eating garlic or onions.[5] Obviously this is no proof but isn't it enticingly suggestive? Why not poll the 13,000 persons in the U.S. known in

---

1. Dickerson, J.W.T., Nutrition, aging and the elderly, Royal Society of Health Journal, April, 1978.
2. Huggins, H.A., Balancing body chemistry for better success in dentistry, J. Preventive Dentistry, Vol. 1, No. 3, Nov./Dec. 1974, 24-27.
3. Cohen, B.J., Dietary factors affecting rats used in aging research, J. Gerontology, Vol. 34, No. 6, 1979, 803-807.
4. Anonymous, Keeping strokes at a distance, The Sciences, Dec. 1979, Vol. 19, No. 10, 4.
5. Anonymous, Centenarians and representatives, Science, Vol. 26, Nov. 30, 1979, 1057.

1979 to be over 100 years of age (compared to 3,200 in 1969) to see what common nutritional denominators there are? Since the over 85 age group is the fastest growing segment of the population why not study this group also?

A common disorder affecting the prostate gland in older men, swelling and inflammation, may be prevented by eating sunflower and pumpkin seeds.[1] (Both seeds contain zinc.) In clinical trials, a daily dose of 50 to 100 milligrams of zinc caused shrinkage of the swollen prostate in 14 of 19 patients and eliminated the need for surgery. Nearly one out of every three elderly men eventually will develop a swollen prostate. We are getting less zinc from our foods today because of excessive food processing; we don't use zinc galvanized cooking utensils anymore; fertilizer reduces the uptake of zinc in plants. Unless we eat food rich in zinc such as sunflower seeds, pumpkin seeds, herring and oysters, on a regular basis, there is a need for diet supplementation. Some vitamin and trace element deficiencies can be spotted by analysis of the chemical content of our hair.[2] Children with systic fibrosis disease have five times the amount of sodium in their hair than others. Only 10 percent of the calcium. There is less sodium than potassium in the hair of those with celiac disease, a disorder of the digestion and utilization of fats. (Usually we have three to four times more sodium than potassium.) Babies suffering from phenylketonuria are below average in magnesium and calcium. Kwashiorkor demonstrates depressed zinc levels. Low chromium content is associated with juvenile-onset diabetes. People with high academic accomplishment seem to show higher hair concentrations than normal of zinc, less iodine, lead, cadmium. Down's syndrome is characterized by low levels of calcium, copper, manganese. Schizophrenic patients evidenced low activity in cadmium and manganese and were high in lead and iron. A disease which manifests itself by

---

1. Anonymous, Sunflower seeds an RX for prostate sufferers, Cincinnati Enquirer, June 30, 1974.
2. Maugh, T., Hair: a diagnostic tool to complement blood serum and urine, Science, Vol. 202, Dec. 22, 1978, 1271-3.

symptons of mental retardation, ataxia telangiectasia, was characterized by small copper concentrations. Zinc is of estimable assistance in the acceleration of wound healing and in improving the tensile strength of the healed surface. The wound exudate is rich in zinc. Topically applied zinc as zinc oxide ointment and zinc sulfate tablets ingested before surgery are effective. Since old people have diminished levels of zinc in their bodies, and since we know they heal more slowly than younger persons, shouldn't a dietary supplementation be called for?

In protracted periods of vitamin C deficiency, there is considerable cholesterol accumulation in the liver.[1] Vitamin C passes rapidly from the plasma into the white cells where it is involved in the immunological defense. It plays a role in liver metabolism, collagen formation and endocrine control. Tissue requirements vary between individuals, depending on age, sex, stress, etc. To maintain tissue saturation in humans, a daily dose of 60 milligrams is recommended.[2] Tissue desaturation of vitamin C may take place during periods of disease and stress such as ulcers, myocardial infarction, atherosclerosis, colds, asthma, anemia, rheumatic fever, rheumatoid arthritis, burns, and cancer. There is an inverse relationship between blood cholesterol levels and tissue vitamin C concentrations. High cholesterol, low vitamin C and vice versa. Sprittle[3] believes atherosclerosis results from a long-term deficiency of vitamin C. Supplementation is called for in this case and also for patients with coronary thrombosis.[4] Rheumatoid arthritis patients should receive 200 milligrams per day of vitamin C, particularly when they are using aspirin.

1. Ginter, E., Vitamin C in lipid metabolism and atherosclerosis, in Vitamin C, Birch, G.G., K. Parker, editors, Halsted Press, Wiley, New York, 1978, 85.
2. Wilson, C.W.D., Vitamin C: Tissue metabolism, over-saturation and desaturation and compensation, in Vitamin C, Birch, G.G., K. Parker, editors, Halsted Press, Wiley, New York, 206.
3. Sprittle, C.R., Lancet, Vol. 2, 1971, 1280.
4. Hume, R., E. Weyers, T. Rowan, D.S. Reid, W.S. Halls, Brit. Heart Journal, Vol. 34, 1972, 238.

Mothers who took supplementary vitamin C during pregnancy had half as many birth deformities in their newborn babies as were found in the control group.[1] We know now that most animals synthesize large amounts of ascorbic acid (vitamin C).[2] The rat makes 26 to 58 milligrams per day for each kilogram of body weight. Several mammals including humans cannot synthesize their own. Blood levels are higher in women than men but are commonly reduced during pregnancy and lactation as well as when oral contraceptives are being used. Old age, cigarette smoking, and aspirin efface our vitamin C levels. So do conditions of stress, high environmental temperatures, burns, fractures, surgery and infection. In 150 surgical patients vitamin C levels dropped by an average of 17 to 20 percent immediately after surgery. Wound reopening occurred eight times as often among patients with low blood levels of vitamin C. By its ability to mobilize certain enzymes that transform fat-soluble compounds into water-soluble ones which are more easily eliminated from the body, vitamin C may help prevent heart attacks and strokes. It becomes easier for us to transport cholesterol deposits to the liver where it is converted to bile. Some believe vitamin C, as an antioxidant, can suppress the cancer-causing activity of nitrites and nitrates used as preservatives in ham, bacon, frankfurters, luncheon meats and smoked fish by preventing the formation of nitrosamines. When fed to animals, it did. The recommended daily allowance of vitamin C is around 45 milligrams each day although 10 milligrams is enough to prevent scurvy. The body pool of vitamin C (the maximum attainable) is approximately 1500 milligrams; the body utilizes about 3 percent of the body pool each day which is how the 45 milligram figure was derived. Survival times of cancer patients with vitamin C therapy are four times that of the control

---

1. Nelson, M.M., J.O. Forfar, Brit. Med. Journal, Vol. 1, 1971, 523.
2. Schneider, M.J., Vitamin C: How much do we need?, The Sciences, Jan.-Feb., 1975, 11-16.

groups.[1] Vitamin C is ineluctably involved with the immune system by increasing the production of lymphocytes under antigen stimulation; it apparently activates the hexose monophosphate shunt system of resting leucocytes. In other words, vitamin C seems to raise the metabolism of these cells. Bacterial killing ability by the leucocytes is seemingly uninfluenced by 200 milligrams of vitamin C but with a ten-fold increase it was significantly impaired, raising a cautionary signal.[2] Malonaldehyde, a product of excess oxidation of polyunsaturated fats has been shown to be carcinogenic and a mutagen on mouse skin and may be neutralized by vitamin C. Among meats, beef seems to generate the highest levels of malonaldehyde; turkey and cooked chicken were next with cheeses registering small concentrations. Vegetables and fruits contained almost none.[3] Vitamin C prevents the worst effects of alcohol and alcoholism—at least in laboratory animals; zinc also was effective.[4] The alcohol content of the blood was found to be significantly lower with vitamin C than in the control group (after repeated alcohol injections for long periods of time).

Since one-third of all elderly males can expect to have prostate troubles, zinc therapy becomes crucial in our aging society. Zinc is also essential in vitamin A metabolism. Chronically low levels of zinc have been reported for those with alcoholic cirrhosis and other liver diseases, tuberculosis, myocardial infarctions, pulmonary infections, Down's syndrome, cystic fibrosis, pregnancy and women taking oral contraceptives. There have been reports of dramatic improvements in patients suffering from leg ulcers and nutritional dwarfism after zinc therapy. The estimated dietary intake of zinc is 10 to 15 milligrams per day while the recommended dosage is 15 milligrams each day. Thus we receive on the average 66 to 100 percent of the recommended daily allowance. It is

---

1. Cameron, E., L. Pauling, Vitamin C and cancer, International Journal of Environmental Studies, Vol. 10, 1977, 303-305.
2. Anonymous, AGE News, Fall, 1977, Vol. 7.
3. Anonymous, AGE News, Spring, 1978, Vol. 8.
4. Anonymous, The advantages of vitamin C, Sunday New York Times, July 3, 1977.

found in seafood, animal meats, eggs, legumes and whole grain. Zinc's presence in animal protein suggests that for the elderly, there may be a difficulty in meeting the minimum daily requirements. The health consequences for the elderly could be less taste acuity and slow wound healing—conditions we do indeed see in the elderly.[1] Surgical wounds in rats rendered zinc deficient had lower tensile strength and healing was delayed. A zinc deficiency impairs RNA metabolism which may obstruct proper synthesis of protein. Zinc sulfate therapy in patients undergoing oral surgery resulted in an improvement in a condition known as "dry sockets"; post tonsillectomy patients were helped; so were those with atherosclerosis. The zinc concentration in wound exudate is two to four times higher than in blood plasma. Zinc sulfate pills successfully treated patients with venus leg ulcers.[2] A zinc deficiency in pregnant rats produced malfunctions in every organ of the young. Even relatively short periods of zinc deficiency produced teratogenicity. Persons suffering from decreased taste acuity (hypogeusic) were found to be low in serum zinc levels, a condition reversed by zinc sulfate therapy.

Vitamin C also is believed to be effective in wound healing, particularly in meeting the post operative stress. (Dogs were more resistant to acute hemorrhage and traumatic shock.) Patients in hemodialysis, on the artificial kidney machine, show a decline in plasma vitamin C concentrations. Atherosclerosis can be engendered in animals by inducing a vitamin C deficiency, even with normal cholesterol readings for the blood. This is reversible by vitamin C therapy. Vitamins C and E influence absorption of iron, Vitamin E also affects the utilization of vitamin A. We need 20 to 30 international units (IU's) of vitamin E daily; the average intake is around 11 IU's. Vitamin E is reported to have

---

1. Greger, J.L., Dietary intake and nutritional status in regard to zinc of institutionalized aged, J. Gerontology, Vol. 32, No. 5, 1977, 549-553.
2. Halsted, J.A., J.C. Smith, Plasma zinc in health and disease, The Lancet, Feb. 4, 1970.

helped children with hemolytic anemia and those suffering nocturnal leg cramps. Persons with Alzheimer's disease show high concentrations of aluminum, silicon and manganese in their brains. Manganese was also high in their serum, hair and feces. Moroccan miners complaining of intermittent low back pain, radiation of pain down the leg and cramping were found to have manganese intoxication.[1] Some of our vitamin and mineral needs are summarized below.[2]

RECOMMENDED DIETARY ALLOWANCES, 1973

	Years	Fat Soluble Vitamins					Water Soluble Vitamins				
		A	D	E	C	Folic Acid	Niacin	Riboflavin	Thiamin	B_6	B_{12}
		I.U.	I.U.	I.U.	mg	mcg	mg	mg	mg	mg	mcg
infants	0-0.5	1400	400	4	35	50	5	0.4	0.3	0.3	0.3
	0.5-1.0	2000	400	5	35	50	8	0.6	0.5	0.4	0.3
children	1-3	2000	400	7	40	100	9	0.8	0.7	0.6	1.0
	4-6	2500	400	9	40	200	12	1.1	0.9	0.9	1.5
	7-10	3300	400	10	40	300	16	1.2	1.2	1.2	2.0
males	11-14	5000	400	12	45	400	18	1.5	1.4	1.6	3.0
	15-18	5000	400	15	45	400	20	1.8	1.5	1.8	3.0
	19-22	5000	400	15	45	400	20	1.8	1.5	2.0	3.0
	23-50	5000		15	45	400	18	1.6	1.4	2.0	3.0
	51+	5000		15	45	400	16	1.5	1.2	2.0	3.0
females	11-14	4000	400	10	45	400	16	1.3	1.2	1.6	3.0
	15-18	4000	400	11	45	400	14	1.4	1.1	2.0	3.0
	19-22	4000	400	12	45	400	14	1.4	1.1	2.0	3.0
	23-50	4000		12	45	400	13	1.2	1.0	2.0	3.0
	51+	4000		12	45	400	12	1.1	1.0	2.0	3.0
pregnant		5000	400	15	60	800				2.5	4.0
lactating		6000	400	15	60	600				2.5	4.0

The rate at which the brain can synthesize the neurotransmitter, acetylcholine can be increased by administering its precursor, choline. Choline or lecithin (the dietary source of choline) is useful in the treatment of tardive dyskinesia, a disease characterized by twitches in facial muscles, rolling tongue, lip smacking, lip puckering, uncontrollable upper trunk movements and rapid eye blinking. About 40 to 50 percent of patients in state mental hospitals have this condition[3], arising as a

---

1. Banta, R.G., W.R. Markesbery, Elevated manganese levels associated with dementia and extrapyramidal signs, Neurology, Vol. 27, March, 1977, 213-216.
2. Food and Nutrition Board, National Academy of Sciences-National Research Council, in Journal of the American Dietic Association, Vol. 64, Feb. 1974, 150.

side effect of their being on the antipsychotic drugs phenothiazine and butyrophenomes. They improve when fed choline; the etiology of the disease is thought to be related to the depletion of acetylcholine in the brain. Choline (or lecithin, a natural choline source) is useful in the treatment of mania and senile dementia, again thought to be caused by a lack of acetylcholine in the brain. Mania patients are usually treated with lithium which can be toxic. Choline treatment of senile dementia

RECOMMENDED DIETARY ALLOWANCES, 1973

Calcium	Phosphorus	Iodine	Iron	Magnesium	Zinc
mg	mg	mcg	mg	mg	mg
360	240	35	10	60	3
540	400	45	15	70	5
800	800	60	15	150	10
800	800	80	10	200	10
800	800	110	10	250	10
1200	1200	130	18	350	15
1200	1200	150	18	400	15
800	800	140	10	350	15
800	800	130	10	350	15
800	800	110	10	350	15
1200	1200	115	18	300	15
1200	1200	115	18	300	15
800	800	100	18	300	15
800	800	100	18	300	15
800	800	80	18	300	15
1200	1200	125	13	450	20
1200	1200	150	13	450	25

(Alzheimer's disease) is not yet regarded as successful. There is an interesting study of the impaired swimming ability of aged rats and the apparent reversal of the problem by feeding the old rats L-dopa, the precursor to dopamine, a neurotransmitter and apomorphine, a dopamine receptor stimulant.[4] Lipofuscin is believed to be implicated in some way in brain dysfunction. Hydergine and centrophenoxine were shown to decrease lipofuscin accumulation in mouse cells.[5] L-dopa, reserpine and

3. Kolata, G.B., Mental disorders: a new approach to treatment?, Science, Vol. 203, Jan. 5, 1979, 36-8.
4. Marshall, J.F., N. Berrios, Movement disorders of aged rats: reversal by dopamine receptor stimulation, Science, Vol. 206, Oct. 26, 1979, 477-9.
5. Nandy, K., F.H. Schneider, Effects of hydergine on aging neuroblastoma cells in culture, Pharmacology, Vol. 16, 1978, 88-92.

chlorpromazine lower body temperature and may therefore in some way extend lifespan.[1] A decrease of core body temperature of 2°C in humans may extend median survival time from 71.8 years to 100 years. Body temperature is regulated by norepinephrine and serotonin levels in the hypothalamus. Rats fed L-dopa showed a 73 percent increase in lifespan. The production of catecholamines, dopamine and norepinephrine (neurotransmitters) are affected by the brain levels of tyrosine, their amino acid precursors.[2]

In starvation (and dieting) our body mobilizes for survival by cutting its oxygen consumption and metabolism.[3] This slowed rate of living and diminished vitality is also characteristic of animals with flaccid thyroids (hypothyroidism). Treating hypothyroidism with thyroxine, the hormone derived from the thyroid, is rendered more difficult—or ineffective—by starvation. Starvation seems to block our response to thyroid hormones such as thyroxine; other thyroid hormone production, triiodothyronine (T3) is also reduced. Voluntary restriction of food intake when young and an ability to maintain a low body temperature in a hot environment tended to be indicative of or actually contributed to a lengthened lifespan for male rats.[4] Reduced food consumption by thermally stressed rats helped increase lifespan more than heat stress shortened it. The rise in rectal temperature of thermally stressed rats was an index of their foreshortened longevity.

Timaras[5] defines one form of aging as the duration of

---

1. Janoff, A.S., B. Rosenberg, Chemically evoked hypothermia in the mouse: towards a method of investigating thermodynamic parameters of aging and death in mammals, Mech. of Aging and Develop., Vol. 3, 1978, 335-349.
2. Wurtman, R.J., Food for thought, The Sciences, Vol. 18, No. 4, April, 1978, 6.
3. Wimpfheimer, C., E. Saville, M.J. Voirol, E. Danforth, A.G. Burger, Starvation-induced decreased sensitivity of resting metabolic rate to triiodothyronine, Science, Vol. 205, Sept. 21, 1979, 1272-3.
4. Kibler, H.H., H.D. Johnson, Temperature and longevity in male rats, Missouri Agricultural Experiment Station, Univ. of Missouri, Columbia, Missouri, Journal Series, No. 2984, 1979, 52-56.
5. Timaras, P.S., Developmental physiology and aging, Macmillan, New York, 1972.

life measured by the time it takes to acquire our mature size: rapid growth, perish sooner. Food restriction experiments have demonstrated this. (In the world of corporations, countries and civilizations—the so-called inanimate systems—industrial development and expansion (differentiation) may imply complexity; baroque complexity could be our clarion call, signaling the onset of decay.) Timaras also characterizes aging in terms of loss of function and cites the example of the blood of a 20-year-old man (which takes up almost 4 liters of oxygen per minute) compared to the 75-year-old man whose blood can only achieve 1.5 liters per minute. He assesses physiologic age by: fecundity (the number of young born each year of adult life is indirectly related to longevity); metabolic rate (shrews have the highest metabolic rate of all mammals); nerve degeneration (the abnormal amounts of lipofuscin accumulated in Batten's disease which displace sphingolipids, resulting in atrophy of the brain of the afflicted children); cellular errors and mutations (lysosomes become less effective in cleaning up the cellular debris in old cells and hence the cells become degraded and toxic substances accumulate); blood red cell degeneration (diminished size, increased cell density, decreased intracellular potassium and increased sodium, reduction in the concentration of the enzyme glucose-6-phosphate dehydrogenase, increased fragility, reduction in surface charge, increased binding together of older red blood cells, changes in the oxygen uptake ability); increased autoimmune diseases (autoantibodies formed against denatured gamma globin deposited in the rheumatoid lesions cause rheumatoid arthritis). Females seem to have a higher incidence of autoimmune diseases than males; immunosuppressant drugs (which dampen our immune function, including the autoimmune response) prolong median survival times of mice.

 Calorically restricted but healthy diets fed to newly-weaned rats increased the maximum lifespan in males.[1]

---

1. Finch, C.E., L. Hayflick, editors, Handbook of the biology of aging, Van Hostrand Reinhold, New York, 1977.

Offspring of young rotifers had longer lifespans than others. Castration in mice leads to longer lifespan; this is true for male cats also. Young rats are three times more responsive to injected thyroxine than old rats. Bovine pituitary extracts can decrease the responsiveness of immature rats to thyroxine. (The death hormone at work?) Hypophysectomy (the removal of the pituitary) in young rats arrests the normal age-associated diminished effect of thyroxine. If done to adults, we find a restoration of their receptivity to thyroxine. (We've removed the source of the death hormone?) Anna Aslan in Rumania treats old people with Gerovital H3 (procaine), which is supposed to inhibit the adrenalin-destroying enzyme MAO (monoamine oxidase), and raise the serotonin level. MAO increases with age.[1] Deanol (dimethylaminoethanol) is used to treat age-related deterioration of brain function by neutralizing the formation of lipofuscin in nerve cells. It is a precursor of choline and acetylcholine. (Choline is added to some multivitamin preparations.) Deanol is believed to work by stabilizing cellular membranes, similar benefits redounding from chlorpromazine, chlorpheniramine, promazine, chlorphenoxamine, and tetracaine. Centrophenoxine, a so-called age retardant is deanol chemically linked with a plant hormone, auxin. Other names for homologous compounds are chlorphenoxine and meclophenoxate, prescribed as normalizers of the central nervous system and as an antidepressant, for mental confusion, apathy, memory defects and fatigue. Animals treated with centrophenoxine exhibited reduced lipofuscin in most parts of the central nervous system. Adding it to the drinking water of senile mice increased their maximum lifespan 25 percent. In Russia, use of Siberian ginseng is supposed to build energy, zest, endurance, stamina, physical and mental ability, improve appetite and sleep. Animals on ginseng lived 20 percent longer than the controls. Vincamine, obtained in Czechoslovakia from the woodland flower periwinkle (genus Vinca) will, if you believe some French

---

1. Hrachovec, J.P., Human life extension, American Laboratory, Oct. 1978, 135-142.

claims, halt or reverse the aging process in our brains by rejuvenating brain cells. Ovulation can be induced in aged female rats by feeding them L-dopa which apparently increases the amount of catecholamines in the hypothalamus, thereby influencing the pituitary.[1] L-dopa is an inhibitor of MAO in the brain and thereby also causes an increase in catecholamines. Removing the spleen apparently improves longevity for aged mice. The spleen is a source of stored T-cells and perhaps by removing the spleen our bodies begin to have access to younger T cells, inducing in effect a more youthful immune system. Injecting young T cells into old rats seems to allow the old rats to survive diseases with fewer fatalities. In general, whatever we can do to limit the monoamine oxidase (MAO) presence will extend lifespan for mammals. Less MAO, more monoamine neurotransmitters and an enhanced nerve transmission system.[2] The ability of brain cells to respond to dopamine (a monoamine) slows with age. Dopamine stimulates the brain receptor enzyme adenylcyclase. And if all else fails, you can always try hypnosis; in one experiment, of 19 women, 35 to 56 years of age, 9 received anti-aging hypnotic suggestions. All nine evidenced a drop in body age three weeks after the hypnosis sessions. The median age loss was 11 years.[3]

---

1. Kurtzman, J., P. Gordon, No more aging, J.P. Tarcher, Los Angeles, 1976.
2. Anonymous, Longlife magazine, Vol. 2, No. 3, July/August, 1978.
3. Morgan, R.F., The adult growth examination, Interamerican Journal of Psychology, Vol. 11, No. 1, 1977, 10-13.

Chapter 15

This You Never Learned In School

Lesson Number 1. The Great Partition Flap

At work they assigned me to a large laboratory, gave me a small desk, the same as all the others. Human traffic in the lab was heavy and therefore distracting as I tried to read or do anything else of substance. Determined to remove myself from the mainstream, I found and put in place two portable room partitioners which effectively sealed off my modest lebensraum from the passersby. Traffic was therefore redirected and redistributed and I was happy. But the corporate powers were disturbed, for it appeared (ominously) that I was constructing for myself a private office, when others had nothing equivalent. It smelled of aggrandisement, they said, and I was ordered to dismantle everything and return to my original condition. Here is the first principle of everyday life: space equals status, status is equivalent to power. Conclusion: space is to be awarded only to the annointed ones.

Lesson Number 2. The Great Right Wing Supervision

We ate lunch together at work, a few of us from the laboratory, collected and led to the cafeteria by our supervisor, the chief of the division. He conducted daily seminars at lunch, excoriating the left wing, including its dupes and sympathizers of liberal causes. Our leader quoted from John Birch Society doctrine and smashed any feeble counter-arguments which arose. Mostly my colleagues sat mute during these lessons from the chairman—who for eight hours a day controlled the work, pay and lives of his underlings. But didn't he also exercise his influence over their private lives, the other sixteen hours of the day? For should he become annoyed with their politics—during the working day— could he not slow their advancement, wouldn't he minimize their pay increments, wasn't he able to fire them from their jobs? Isn't the question rhetorical, didn't he really control their whole lives, not just the eight-hour block? So my group sat in silence—except for me. My courage grew only after I had an academic job in hand. Then I was able to break the siege and question our supervisor openly, challenging his promulgated hypotheses. I bore the brunt of his diatribes until I departed to pursue my greater love, an academic career. Thus I learned the second principle of everyday life: he who works for money is never free. Conclusion: work for yourself, for the satisfaction of it and for the benefit of your family and mankind. Second conclusion: this is an unattainable idealism for most of us.

Lesson Number 3. Henry in the Shithouse

As a rookie at work, I had assigned to me an old fellow called Henry, who as a technician, was to assist in my experimental work. Henry was close to retirement, had a strong union and was almost always to be found in the lavatory. Shithouse Henry, he was called and he was going to help me. We began, as others had begun with Henry, and nothing was getting done. Henry was in top form. But then, I hit upon it, one of those original, useful ideas which change the world: why not erect a sign, prominently displayed, on our budding equipment. It would announce the title of the project along with our names, Henry's and mine, equal in size and rank. It was done, and the results were close to miraculous. Shithouse Henry became a human dynamo, working long hours effectively, pushing me steadily, urging us to succeed. And we did, thanks largely to Henry who now had recognition and satisfaction. Thus I learned the third principle of everyday life: recognition, like love is boundless.

Conclusion: it never hurts to love a little more and to share your fame and success and prestige. In love and esteem, one plus one can equal three and no one gets hurt.

Lesson Number 4. The Tea Party

Way back in ancient history, when universities were ivory towers and professors were eggheads, little old spinster Deans gave teas for the daughters of the alumni who were sent by their parents to their alma mater. Though this was not ancient history, nevertheless my Department Head gave a tea at his home for the new faculty members in the Department.

Mrs. Head was pouring as they say in the society columns.

"Would you like some tea?"

Under such social conditions, I was no tea drinker. She's got to be kidding. In this day and age this lady is pushing tea?

When a lady sticks her body next to yours and offers you some tea, its hard to refuse. I furtively searched in vain for the alcoholic drinks while I stalled. Slowly I adjusted my glasses while maintaining a frozen smile on my face.

"What have you got?" I asked her, still looking for help.

"Oh, what a question! We've got five different kinds of tea: Orange Pekoe; Cut Black; Oolong; Gun Powder Green and Souchang Black."

I mumbled some choice of tea, collected a few sterile cookies to neutralize the tea and retreated from the party. I explored the house and returned after a while to the living room where everyone was seated in a circle. The chairs and sofas being occupied, I propped myself against a wall, tea in hand and locked my knees in place. Soon Nictus and Hervae Gobbloy approached and very formally Nictus introduced himself and his wife.

"This is my wife, Hervae", said Dr. Nictus Gobbloy. "Mrs. Gobbloy is really Dr. Gobbloy also, since she has a

Ph.D. So we are really Dr. and Dr. Nictus and Hervae Gobbloy."

Nictus was a full professor, a senior member of the Department and was now coming on very strong. Nictus volunteered that he got his Ph.D. in 1940 and was knowledgeable in my area of interest. All this was seemingly said in one long breath as I stood mute. Was all this verbiage overcompensation, politics or genuine good will? It was obvious that lathered in amidst all the words was a bit of self praise and some old fashioned intimidation.

"Oh, isn't that interesting," I mumbled finally.

Bully for you, I thought. Nictus also told of his wonderfully talented children as I stood sponge-like in the corner and absorbed this startling information. Fourth Principle of Everyday Life: anyone who drinks tea when alcoholic beverages are called for should be invisible. Conclusion: sterile cookies generate sterile people.

Lesson Number 5. The Departmental Meeting

The Department assembled for the first faculty meeting of the year, with Doctor Head at the head of the table. Head commenced the meeting by making some trivial announcements, mentioning things that were already common knowledge. There was extensive discussion of the trivia; the major contributors to these vacuous debates seemed to be Nictus Gobbloy and Sash Cestort. Nictus referred to everyone with a Ph.D. as "Doctor", those with less than this exalted degree he called "Professor" or "Mister".

"Doctor Cestort, I disagree with your idea that we ought to stock green paper as well as traditional white paper in the toilets," Nictus pronounced gravely.

"Surely you are aware of the psychological effects that the color green has on bodily functions," said Dr. Gobbloy, authoritatively.

"That may be so," responded Dr. Cestort, "but the color variations are important in an educational institution in order to teach the students how to discriminate and make decisions."

I observed a very curious phenomenon during this exchange and the subsequent ones. Autocatalysis. For example (using a chemistry example), as a chemical reaction yields a certain product, the speed of the reaction increases as the product is accumulated. This is autocatalysis. Thus as the product is generated, the reaction gets faster, giving more product, giving a still faster reaction, etc. Nictus Gobbloy was autocatalytic! He began by speaking slowly (the reaction). As he heard his own words, these words (the product) seemed to generate in him more enthusiasm for his monologue, which of course resulted in more words, which gave him more spirit to go on, yielding more words, etc. There surely would have been a "verbular" explosion except for the fact that Sash Cestort had the finesse to interrupt the process. Unfortunately, Sash was also autocatalytic and could only be interrupted by Nictus. The Fifth Principle of Everyday Life: one should always take green toilet paper into a departmental faculty meeting. Conclusion: a professor who talks too much could destroy the world.

Lesson Number 6. Just Who The Hell Do They Think They Are? (1958)

You give an inch and they try to take a mile. You build some schools for them and are they satisfied? No Sir! And are they grateful? To hell they are! Well if they want to play rough we'll show them who's boss. They'll realize how good they had it when they didn't get in our way— and to hell with the Supreme Court. Those bunch of Communists sitting there taking orders from the Jews— and the next thing you know we'll have a Catholic in the White House and then the country will really go to the dogs.

I can't understand why they're making all the fuss about eating at those lunch counters. It's probably orders from those Communists in the N.A.A.C.P. who are filling them full of phony ideas of freedom and equality. They're free here and happy. Don't we give them jobs as porters and bus boys? What's wrong with good honest work? They wouldn't be happy doing any job that needs thinking. You know they can't. It's up to us Whites to take care of them.

We had pretty good race relations before those Yankees filled their heads full of Communist ideas. We got a southern way of life to protect—which is pretty damn good—and nobody, white, black, yellow or any of those other colors is going to force us to change. And besides, it's God's will to have things just as they are, the Bible says so.

And besides, it's a states rights issue and we've got some real scrappers in Congress who are all for us. It don't matter what the Bill of Rights says, or what the socialist, Lincoln, said. We got the right to do what we please—it's part of our civil rights and liberty—that's why America is so great.

Next thing you know they'll be sitting next to us in the airport waiting rooms, and then in our schools—big, black boys next to our pretty, white girls—and God, what next— they'll be marrying our girls and raising a mongrel race. By God that's not going to happen here! Everybody knows the white race is the best—and a pure strain too, like a thoroughbred. And that's the way we're going to keep it. Who the hell do they think they are anyway?

Lesson Number 7. If Both the Negro and White Beliefs in God are Valid, Then It Can Be Shown That There Are Two Gods: A Negro and A White (1959)

Consider the all-White congregations of all-White churches. Certainly these congregations require White preachers to enlighten them and interpret God's will.

Since by hypothesis the Negro belief in God is held to be valid, then the Negro people too must have revelation. They gather in congregations to absorb God's message from Negro preachers in Negro churches.

Because mortal man never outgrows his need for divine guidance, so it is reasonable to assume that when he dies, his soul, if it is worthy, will ascend to heaven and again seek communion with God. Thus both Negro and White ascend upon death to the glorious eternity of heaven.

If man is made in God's image, so also is his ecclesiastic structure and hence, in heaven, the immortal souls of man gather in congregations to worship. Here also there must be White congregations, preached to by White angels and Negro congregations, preached to by Negro angels. Since the angels also require revelation, the White angels must gather in White congregations and the Negro angels gather in Negro congregations. Certainly, there must be a White preacher for the White congregation of angels and this would be the greatest preacher of them all; none other than God himself. Of course he is White. For the Negro congregation of angels there must be a Negro preacher; the highest preacher of them all, the Negro God.

It can be easily shown that the Negro God and the White God represent the highest order of divinity.

Suppose that there is a still higher order of divinity. Then this supreme God must also preach to a congregation—in this case the congregation consists of only the Negro God and the White God. However, this leads to a contradiction, since Negro and White cannot be present in the same congregation. Hence our supposition of a single supreme God is invalidated.

Thus, there must be two Gods, a Negro God and a White God.

Chapter 16

Energy, Entropy, Exercise, Basal Metabolism and Lifespan

Life is a series of chemical reactions accelerated or moderated and modulated by enzymes. We store or expend energy by this route and if we are constant temperature beings—as we are—then we transfer to the surroundings most of the resulting energy as heat, generated by the metabolism of fats, carbohydrates and protein. Fats are insoluble, transported in the blood, bound to protein as lipoprotein. They may be triglycerides, derived from fatty acids and glycerol. Fats in foodstuffs and fatty deposits in animals consist of mixtures of triglycerides. Some typical fatty acids are palmitic and stearic acids (saturated or solid fatty acids) and the unsaturated or liquid fatty acids such as linoleic acid (found in vegetable oils) and arachidonic acid (in fish and animals). Fats, when absorbed, circulate to the liver where as triglycerides they are hectored into becoming fatty acids. From the liver the fats pass into the blood and then to adipose tissue for storage. Blood triglyceride levels are increased by fats high in saturated fatty acids such as beef fat and butter. Thyroid hormones and physical exercise diminish their presence. From adipose tissue fats are carried to muscle where they are oxidized to carbon dioxide and water to yield energy. Fat utilization is enhanced by adrenalin and noradrenalin and growth hormone from the pituitary. Emotional stimuli increase fat mobilization.

Sugars and starches (carbohydrates) are absorbed as glucose. Insulin secretion is stimulated by glucose; glucose moves via the bloodstream to nerve tissue where it is oxidized to release the energy required for neuron function. And to muscle, to be stored as glycogen or oxidized to produce energy or converted into fat when in excess. Glycogen can be reactivated by conversion to glucose by adrenalin. If done rapidly without sufficient oxygen (anaerobically), lactic acid is produced. In starvation, when no carbohydrate is available, the energy of life comes from fat, changed in the liver to "ketone bodies", acetone and other substances, most of which are eliminated in the urine. Insulin facilitates the passage of glucose through the cell wall. Adrenalin produces a rise in blood glucose by releasing it from the liver. Caffeine raises the blood glucose level.[1] Protein can be oxidized in the liver for energy (producing urea).

In our cells immediate energy flows from the breakdown of adenosine triphosphate (ATP) to adenosine diphosphate (ADP) by the reaction of glucose and ATP to yield glucose-6-phosphate plus ADP. Heat is liberated, serving to maintain normal body temperature. Exercising after a meal will approximately double our body's heat generation (measured as the basal metabolic rate, the heat transferred from the body to the ambient air under carefully controlled resting conditions).[2] The metabolic rate may increase in response to a cold environment, on the order of 10 to 30 percent.

Metabolizing vegetable and fish oils (with polyunsaturated fatty acids) effectively lowers cholesterol levels; the opposite is true for animal fats (saturated fatty acids). Large meals lead to higher levels of fatty materials in the blood and has the effect of boosting the net caloric content in the food.[3] One large meal in the evening can be devastating in its effect. Basal metabolic rates (BMR) measurements seem to vary by 10 percent during the day. Overfeeding can raise the BMR by 29 percent; underfeeding can drop it by 17 percent. The BMR is defined as the energy output of an individual under standardized resting conditions: bodily and mentally at rest; 12 to 18

---

1. Cheraskin, E., Effect of caffeine versus placebo supplementation in blood glucose correlations, Lancet, Vol. 1, 1967, 1299.
2. Miller, D.S., P. Mumford, Obesity, physical activity and nutrition, Proc. Nutr. Soc., Vol. 25, 1966, 100.
3. Bray, G.A., Lipogenesis in human adipose tissue, J. Clinical Invest., Vol. 51, 1972, 537.

hours after a meal; in a thermally neutral environment. Strictly speaking circadian rhythms affect the basal metabolic rate and should also be factored into the experimental conditions arranged when doing BMR measurements. Minor disturbances in the testing room can cause alarums and an 11 percent change in the BMR. The effect of changes in deep body temperature on metabolic rate is quite well established: a 1°C rise caused by fever or other means translates into a 12 percent increase in BMR. Similarly, the effect of hypothermia (lowering the body temperature) in reducing the metabolic rate is well known; use is made of this in some surgical procedures. The basal metabolic rate decreases during undernutrition, to a greater extent than mere loss of body weight can explain; resumption of feeding restores the metabolic rate to normal long before body weight achieves its initial value. Should the subject again be underfed, the metabolic rate now falls more rapidly than before. High protein diets have a thermal effect, that is, they raise the BMR; fats and carbohydrates do also, but to a lesser degree. In obese persons on diets, there is a more rapid loss of weight if they are fed their equivalent calories in smaller, more frequent doses. As obese people lose weight their BMR drops; they may have BMR values lower than the rest of the population and therefore, even while eating normally may continue to maintain an overweight condition.

It has been estimated that on the average we spend 8 hours a day in bed, 50 to 60 percent of our leisure time sitting and out of the whole day, only 3 to 9 percent of our energy and time standing.[1] BMR values tend to reach a minimum during the summer months and a maximum in the winter for some Japanese and Korean men.[2] Energy expenditures at rest and during physical exercise in a thermally neutral environment are greater in winter than in summer. People of tropical countries, Scandanavians and those from Singapore have lower BMR values in

---

1. Shock, N.W., The physiology of aging, Scientific American, No. 1, Jan., 1962, 100-109.
2. Gold, A.J., A. Zornitzer, S. Samueloff, Influence of season and heat on energy expenditure during rest and exercise, J. Appl. Physiology, Vol. 27, No. 1, 1969, 9-12.

general than equivalent persons from the Western world.[1]

With advancing age there is a progressive decrease in the power of the heart to adapt to exertion and stress. Although resting blood pressure in healthy individuals increases only slightly with age, a given amount of exercise will raise heart rate and blood pressure in old people more than it will in young.[2] During exercise, the old heart is less able to increase stroke volume and the blood vessels are less able to accept increased amounts of blood. This imposes limits on the amount of work the elderly can do. Activity is also affected by a decline in respiratory function. There is a loss in mechanical efficiency resulting from musculoskeletal changes. Chest measurements decrease during the transition from ages forty-five to eighty-five and the thoracic cage becomes more rigid, thus inhibiting expansion. The alveoli enlarge and thin out and bronchioles lose elasticity. The diaphragm becomes fibrotic and weakened, lessening its efficiency. An emphysema-like condition is seen to develop.[3] The amount of oxygen the blood takes up from the lungs and transports to the tissues during exercise falls substantially with age.

In order to double the oxygen uptake during exercise, the older individual must move about 50% more air in and out of his lungs. A decline in arterial oxygen saturation reflects in part the reduced heart output: less blood flows through the lungs of the older person in a given time period. Vital capacity (the amount of air that can be forcibly expired from the lung) diminishes with age and the maximum breathing capacity (the amount of air that can be moved through the lungs in 15 seconds) shows a decline of about 40% between the ages of twenty and eighty.[4] The older person cannot maintain as fast a rate of

1. Banerjee, B., N. Saka, Energy cost of some common daily activities for active tropical male and female subjects, J. Appl. Physiology, Vol. 29, No. 2, 1970, 200-3.
2. Birren, J.E., R.N. Butler, S.W. Greenhouse, L. Sokoloff, M.R. Yarrow, Human aging: A biological and behavioral study, Washington, D.C., U.S. Printing Office for NIH, 1963.
3. DeBeauvoir, S., The coming of age, G.P. Putnam, 1973.
4. Shock, N.W., The physiology of aging, Scientific American, Jan., 1962, 106-109.

breathing as a younger person. Because the heart pumps less blood with advancing age, less blood flows through the kidney. Changes within the kidney itself further reduce the flow of blood as well as the efficiency with which the kidney processes bodily wastes. Tests of kidney function show that between the ages of thirty-five and eighty the flow of blood through the kidney declines by 55 per cent. Filtration rate and excretory capacity decline to the same extent. Reduction in blood flow through the kidney is apparently an adaptive mechanism since it seems to result from construction of kidney blood vessels, making more blood available for other organs. The kidney of the older person has less blood to work on and requires more time to perform its functions.

There are questions raised, whether activity can add productive years to our lifespan and can activity protect us from the pathological signs of old age. Some believe exercise, when extended over a lifetime will prolong the active years.[1] A Duke University study, an activity inventory dealing with participation in family, work, health, religious and leisure activities was administered to a group over sixty years of age. It was found that high activity scores correlated with absence of disability.[2] The relationship between exercise and clinical symptoms was further demonstrated in a study using the Cornell Medical Health Index Questionnaire. The prevalence of pathology was significantly higher in both younger and older groups who had no daily exercise, but was even more sharply defined in the older group. In early life the body is endowed with tremendous reserve capacities. The loss of a few hundred cells hardly affects the performance of an organ. According to Selye, eventually the stress of living imposes demands beyond the capacity of the organism: aging depends largely on the rate of wear and tear, for life

---

1. Edington, D.W., A. Cosmos, W.B., McCafferty, Exercise and longevity, evidence for threshold age, J. Gerontology, Vol. 27, No. 3, 1972, 341-3.
2. Jeffers, F., C.R. Nichols, The relationship of activities and attitudes to physical well-being in older people, in Normal aging, Report of the Duke longevity study, 1955-1969, E. Palmore, editor, Durham, N.C., Duke University Press, 1970, 304-318.

is essentially a process which gradually spends the given amount of adaptive energy that we inherited from our parents.[1] Selye compared vitality to a bank account from which we can make withdrawals but cannot increase by deposits. And the only control over this is the rate at which one makes withdrawals.

Hanson, et.al.[2] conducted a seven month physical training program on 25 normal 40 to 49 year-old men. The study revealed that physical conditioning can produce lowered heart rates at rest and after treadmill exercises. Stamford[3] studied the effects of training on institutionalized patients. The nine patients in the experimental group had a mean age of 71.5 years and the control group's mean age was 65.2 years. Stamford found that results of tests performed on a bicycle ergometer and a motor-driven treadmill produced a mean heart rate decrease of eight beats per minute. Pollock[4] conducted a study with 16 men (mean age 48.9) to determine the effects of walking on body composition and cardiovascular functioning. He found that maximal O_2 uptake was increased, pulmonary ventilation was increased, the diastolic blood pressure at rest was decreased, and the heart rate during exercise decreased from 4 to 17 beats per minute. In the same study, there was a reduction in total body weight and fat. There was a greater utilization of oxygen in the muscle tissue of a physically trained person regardless of age.[5] The effects of exercise on joint stiffness was studied to determine to what extent stiffness was a function of aging and to what extent was it activity-

---

1. Selye, H., The stress of life, N.Y., McGraw-Hill, 1950.
2. Hanson, J.S., B.S. Tabakin, A.M. Levy, W. Nedde, Long term physical training and cardiovascular dynamics in middle-aged men, Circulation, Vol. 38, Nov. 1968, 783-799.
3. Stamford, B.A., Physiological effects of training upon institutionalized geriatric men, J. Gerontology, Vol. 27, Nov. 4, 1972, 451-5.
4. Pollock, M.L., H.S. Miller, R. Janeway, A.C. Linnerud, R. Robertson, R. Valentine, Effects of walking on body composition and cardiovascular function of middle-aged men, J. Appl. Physiol., Vol. 30, No. 1, 1971, 126-130.
5. Bergman, H., P. Bjorntorp, B. Conradson, M. Toklen, J. Stenberg, E. Varnauskas, Enzymatic and circulating adjustments to physical training in middle-aged men, European, J. Clin. Invest., No. 3, 1973, 414-8.

dependent.[1] After the training program joint stiffness in both old and young were shown to be a reversible process. The question of what happens to collagen during exercise was examined by Faris.[2] He concluded that the collagen found in rat tail tendon can be broken down by temperature changes and acidemia, both of which occur when one exercises. With age we lose our capacity for work but the decline need not be so drastic if we are in good physical condition. Sedentary elderly persons suffer a decline of 31 percent in maximum oxygen uptake but for the active old, this loss is only 10 percent.[3] Good conditioning can be achieved by exercise which stresses the heart at 40 percent of its maximum capacity. Institutionalized geriatric mental patients training at a 50 percent of maximum heart rate level for 18 weeks were able to improve their physical condition. Twenty-two persons confined in bed for six days had elevated concentrations of urinary nitrogen, reduced oxygenation capability and took one to two weeks to recover their lost functions. Deconditioning can raise the heart rate by 25 beats per minute and diminish maximum oxygen uptake by 27 percent.

The elderly may not live longer by physical conditioning but at least by being active they can attempt to avoid the symptoms of stagnation such as low esteem, fear of competition, even fear of success. Some old people say time is short, too short to start another life and try alternative roads. There is a fear of obsolescence (we cannot admit that what we are doing is no longer good enough). We need to practice successful aging, to stay in training in an intellectual and devotional sense. For many old persons, successful aging is directly related to a living spouse.

---

1. Chapman, E.A., H.A. deVries, R. Swezly, Joint stiffness effects of exercise on old and young, J. Gerontology, Vol. 27, No. 2, 1972, 218-22.
2. Faris, A.W., The effects of physical training upon the collagen content of the aorta of adult male white rats, J. Sports Medicine and Physical Fitness, Vol. 13, No. 2, 1973, 108-110.
3. Bassey, E.J., Age, inactivity and some physiological responses to exercise, Gerontology, vol. 24, 1978, 66-77.

Calisthenics, swimming or jogging affect the cardiorespiratory system equally. The average lifespan of athletes seems to be about the same as the general population. For athletes, the order of increasing longevity is: football players; boxers; baseball players and track and field competitors who live the longest. Exercise may not reverse the impairments of old age but we may fervently hope there is some amelioration of the decrepitude we see in our brains: small arterioles with thickened walls containing an amyloid (yellow) old age pigment; the cortex or outer layer shrunken in appearance; a decreased cell count; a loss of weight; lipofuscin (brown) old age deposits; an increase in water content; protein loss; a diminished level of vitamin C.

We, you and I, birds and mammals, maintain constant body temperature by metabolic means. Usually our body temperatures are set above ambient conditions.[1] On the other hand, reptiles and fish assume the temperature of the environment, their metabolic processes just sufficient to maintain life but not able to fix an isothermal body temperature. We (mammals and birds) require 5 to 10 times more energy to live than reptiles of similar size and body temperature. The resting heart rates of 18 species of spiders range from 9 to 125 beats per minute, a function of body size. It mimics the BMR. For the spider, the BMR is 2.5 times the resting heart rate.[2] We search for the measures of aging, the factors affecting it and which characterize our isomorphism. In examining the question of how long we live, we need to face one monumental misconception. Figures are bandied about, as to the length of life of the human species. We speak in terms of life expectancy and report that for males this has climbed to 65 and 70; for females life expectancy is in the seventies. These statements are misleading for the numbers represent the average life expectancy, taking into account the early deaths in infancy, by accident and the myriad of other causes. Naturally life expectancy increases as

---

1. Bennet, A.F., J.A. Ruben, Endothermy and activity in vertebrates, Science, Vol. 206, Nov. 9, 1979, 649-653.
2. Carrel, J.E., R.D. Heathcote, Heart rate in spiders: influence of body size and foraging energetics, Science, Vol. 193, July 9, 1976, 148-150.

medicine progresses and we find more ways to maintain the life of infants and cure diseases of the young. There is another angle to this, in that we can calculate the additional years of expected life, as a function of the age already achieved. For example, at age 55, how many years of life should you expect to achieve, based on the data already available on those 55 and over? The answer may surprise you: we can expect to live way beyond the 70 years that's been quoted so liberally. What we seek is the ultimate lifespan, that age we would achieve if we proceeded to a senile death, uncomplicated by sudden death or catastrophic illness. To find these ages, the table below[1] is useful.

Age	Additional Years of Life		Life Expectancy	
	Male	Female	Male	Female
45	28.4	34.5	73.4	79.5
50	24.2	30.1	74.2	80.1
55	20.4	25.8	75.4	80.8
60	16.8	21.8	76.8	81.8
65	13.7	18.0	78.7	83.0
70	10.9	14.4	80.9	84.4
75	8.6	11.2	83.6	86.2
80	6.8	8.7	86.8	88.7
85	5.3	6.6	90.3	91.6

As we get older, 60, 65, 70, 75, 80, 85 . . . , the additional years of life get smaller and smaller, but at the same time life expectancy reaches higher and higher, aiming for the ultimate life expectancy, that age where additional years shrinks to nothing. In other words, extrapolating from 65 to beyond age 85, we seek that age for males where additional years goes from 13.7 to 10.9, 8.6, 6.8, 5.3..., to 0.0. We discover by this procedure that the ultimate lifespan for males is 103 years and 110 years for females.[2] Faced with these numbers, we need to develop a renascent view of age, especially old age. It would seem that middle age should now include the 60's, then we evolve as young-old,

---
1. Anonymous, Statistical Bulletin of the Metropolitan Life Insurance Company, Vol. 59, No. 3, July-Sept., 1978, 9.
2. Hershey, D., H.H. Wang, A new age-scale for humans, Lexington Books, D.C. Heath, Lexington, 1980.

middle-old and finally old-old (about age 90). We seek the knowledge to enable our population to remain in reasonably good health into young-old age. Thereafter the deracinations of middle-old age become pronounced and it becomes simply a matter of keeping the old-old comfortable and in a decent frame of mind. We can do this by supporting the many-facted aspects of research—wherever they may lead—allowing sufficient time and funding for intelligent and compassionate minds to assimilate the new information and attach some coherency to it.

For 11 years the Russians have been injecting into middle aged and elderly persons human placenta serum. They claim blood pressure dropped, the flow of blood to the brain improved, blood sugar levels went down, sexual function was restored—even in 90 year elders. Memory and agility were reinvested, reflexes quickened and eyesigns strengthened: even an improved resistance to common illnesses.[1] Whatever is in the placenta—we can assume it is rich in the hormones which stimulate our essential functions—nothing has yet to be published by the Russians detailing exactly what are the active ingredients in the placenta serum. What can we say except the usual, trite "more research needs to be done...". As people grow older, they report that the days, months and years seem to be passing more rapidly; a year seems shorter at 60 than at 10 years of age.[2]

Calisthenics, swimming and jogging we know are good for us.[3] Is there a relationship between exercise and a treatment for leukemia? B cell lymphocytes obtained from mice donors when immunized with myeloma cell extract yield antibodies which when injected into leukemic mice seem beneficial in the treatment of leukemia.[4] Combined

---

1. Gris, H., Scientists halt aging process, National Enquirer, Oct. 18, 1972, 28.
2. Walker, J.L., Time estimation and total subjective time, Perceptual and Motor Skills, Vol. 44, 1977, 527-532.
3. Joseph, J.J., Effects of calisthenics, jogging and swimming on middle-aged men, J. Sports Medicine, Vol. 14, 1974, 14-20.
4. Bernstein, I.D., M.R. Tam, R.C. Nowinski, Mouse leukemia therapy with monoclonal antibodies against a thymus differentiation antigen, Science, Vol. 207, Jan. 4, 1980, 68-71.

with an exercise program, would this procedure yield dramatically improved results? Can we do this for humans? Who will be our guinea pigs?

There are claims that the lifespan of mammals is related to brain size and the lifetime accumulation of metabolic activity (the total heat evolved or the energy expended in the course of living).[1] Calloway[2,3] hypothesizes that there is a fixed amount of bodily heat generation potential available in the vicinity of death and that this may be a universal characteristic of living tissue, independent of species. And this constant may be 20 kilocalories per kilogram weight per day. In other words, with time our vitality diminishes until a critical plateau is reached when there is not sufficient energy to maintain life. And so we die. That minimum critical level of heat production in our bodies is the same for you and me and horses, pigs and ants. Survival curves for fruit flies, viruses and bacteria behave similarly. What we find generally is that survival curves look the same, projecting a universal aspect to dying, whether it is individual cells, multicellular agglomerates such as the organs of our bodies or automobiles or houses. Now the real work is to begin, more difficult yet exquisitely intriguing: to search for those unifying principles common to the life process and its unwinding. Are we also to be ineluctably drawn to countries and civilizations? Islam is just under 1,400 years old, Christianity is getting on towards 2,000 and Buddhism was born 2,600 years ago.[4] As living entities, religions have their own morphology and should not, therefore, be strangers to the waning powers of middle and old age. According to Jansen, in the year 1400 A.D. the Christian Church was the most powerful and vital force in what had become its European homeland. On the

---

1. Sacher, G.A., Longevity, aging and death: an evolutionary perspective. The Gerontologist, Vol. 18, No. 2, 1970, 112-119.
2. Calloway, N.O., A critical ratio of aging: water loss-heat production, J. Amer. Geriatrics Society, Vol. 19, No. 5, 1971, 386-390.
3. Calloway, N.O., Heat production and senescence, J. Amer. Geriatric Soc. Vol. 22, No. 4, 1974, 149-150.
4. Jansen, G.H., Militant Islam. The historical whirlwind, The New York Times magazine, Jan. 6, 1980, 14-18.

other hand, Buddhism by 800 A.D. (the 1400th year of its life) was showing signs of old age, though it was still widely practiced throughout India. Is Islam now in its vigorous early middle life, retracing the history of other religions? Kohr[1] proposes that when a society grows beyond its optimum size, human facilities and political systems are overwhelmed. The problem is not to grow but to stop growing. Kohr's answer is not union but division.

Systems, living and otherwise are highly improbable and complex, composed of subsystems, organs, tissue, cells and processes. The human system involves a consanguity of 60 trillion cells.[2] Constant work and energy expenditures are required to keep them in their proper places. Some imperfections always remain. At first these imperfections are subtle and unnoticeable on a microscopie level; with time, however, more and more cells are not restored to their original conditions or configurations after some dislocation or stress. These imperfections gradually accumulate until a weak spot occurs in a vital organ leading ultimately to the collapse of the entire system. How long can a body survive with the continuous development of imperfections? This depends upon our environment, heredity, life style, nutrition and mental state. We could be done in by a decreasing efficiency of the respiratory circulatory subsystem which starves portions of the brain of oxygen and nutrients and hence causes dysfunctions. Part of the explanation of why we age is the stochastic, random and probabilistic nature of the process of living. The errors induced are also attributed to the effects of entropy, a concept borrowed from thermodynamics, a discipline studied by chemists, engineers and those interested in information theory. Entropy is a measure of the availability of energy and its information content. Highly ordered systems carry low entropy and much stored infor-

---

1. Kohr, L., The breakdown of nations, Dutton, New York, 1979. Development without aid, Schocken, New York, 1979. The overdeveloped nations, Schocken, New York, 1979.
2. Samaras, T.T., The law of entropy and the aging process, Human Development, Vol. 17, 1974, 314-320.

mation. Entropy can be defined as a measure of the disorder or randomness of a system engaged in spontaneous actions; it predicts that the system when left to itself inevitably deteriorates with time until its increasing state of disorder achieves a maximum (synonymous with death, the ultimate state of disorder). If the death of an organism is viewed as the state characterized by maximum disorder and if the wear and tear theory offers one reasonable explanation of our longevity, then it should be informative to determine the total entropy production during our lifetimes. Comparisons of the lifetime entropy production for rats, dairy cattle, mules, horses, guinea pigs and humans were estimated[1]; the resulting numbers were quite close, of the same order of magnitude except for humans who were 4 to 5 times higher. From this questions can be asked, such as: Is the lifetime entropy accumulation the same for all animals? Can a new age-scale be defined based on these ideas? Why are humans different?

For living systems, our energy content, entropy production, vitality and rate of living are enmeshed with the chemical reactions within our bodies, affected by temperature. The heat evolved, measured under proper conditions is called the basal metabolic rate (BMR). For each of us there is an internal temperature at which we are comfortable; above this, vasodilation and active sweating occurs; below the set-point vasoconstriction and increased metabolism due to shivering is called for. Under fasting conditions (no food for 12 to 14 hours) and at rest (subject lying quietly under no overt stress), the energy of living is converted almost entirely into heat rejected to our surrounding environment. Astronauts—men and women—living in a space habitat with gravity at 50 to 75 percent of that on earth exhibited lower metabolic rates for reasons still obscure except perhaps for the fact that less energy was required to properly maintain muscle tone in outer space than on earth where gravity is more of a

---

1. Hershey, D., Entropy, basal metabolism and life expectancy, Gerontologia, Vol 7, 1963, 245-250.

factor pressing in on us.[1] And will this diminished metabolic rate reward space travelers with a longer lifespan? Cancer patients record higher metabolic rates than normal despite their significantly curtailed caloric intake. Those suffering cardiovascular disease are likewise hypermetabolic.[2] A group of 50 smokers were found to be experiencing greater sleep difficulties than a group of 50 nonsmokers matched by age and sex.[3] Sleep patterns significantly improved when the smokers abstained. Smoking raises blood pressure, heart rate and fatty acid concentrations. Withdrawal is accompanied by mood and behavioral changes such as depression, lack of concentration, irritation, anxiety, tension and restlessness. For smokers the BMR is elevated, confirming the suspicion that smokers are on some sort of "high", living at an accelerated pace and are physiologically older than their chronological age would indicate. And probably they will suffer shortened lifespans if you believe the wear and tear (rate of living) theory of aging. This effect on the BMR may explain why smokers who kick the habit gain weight. It's true that they in abstinence seek another form of oral gratification and find it in eating. It is also true that their taste buds recover from the noxious chemical contacts which seemed to shrivel and deactivate them. What may be the controlling factor in the rapid weight gain when smokers cease lighting up their cigarettes probably can be understood in relation to the BMR, which is elevated while the subjects are active smokers. The diet of smokers, adequate to maintain a constant weight (when the BMR is high) becomes too rich in calories when the smoking ceases. BMR values drop and now the diet which was sufficient to maintain a fixed girth yields too many calories (the BMR is depressed—or returned to normal) and unless the ex-smoker reduces the amount of food consumed, he or she might gain weight.

1. Economos, A.C., Space gerontology: Altered gravity as a gerontological research tool, presented at the 31st meeting of the Gerontology Society, Dallas, Nov. 1978.
2. Tzankoff, S.P., A.H. Norris, Longitudinal changes in basal metabolism in men, J. Appl. Physiol., Vol. 45, 1978, 536-9.
3. Soldatos, C.R., J.D. Kales, M.B. Scharf, E.O. Bixler, A. Kales, Cigarette smoking associated with sleep difficulty, Science, Vol. 207, Feb. 1, 1980, 551-3.

Biological processes may be cyclical.[1] Some biological rhythms approximate the motif of the seasons, others adhere to the constraints of the lunar month and tides and still others to the 24-hour day. Renal function, enzyme activity, running patterns in rodents, susceptibility to drugs and insecticides, body temperatures and endocrine secretions are examples of daily rhythmic phenomena. Not all of these diurnal rhythms are dependent only on periodic environmental changes in light and temperature but may also be linked to one or more endogenous factors (internal pacemakers). Urine and body temperature can be affected by an abnormally lighted ambience. Perhaps aging is a result of a loss of coordination among many interdependent oscillating systems within our bodies. With advancing age, cyclic processes in different organs become increasingly dissociated. The ultimate loss of function may proceed in multistep fashion where each stage is affected by the preceding one.[2] Or is it a bit more complicated and not so linear; we are all dependent folks, everything growing within and on us. What one subsystem does affects another. If time seems to fly more rapidly with age as has been reported (dependent upon our lifetime accumulation and intensity of experiences) can we allow that the cells of our bodies are likewise influenced by their own, unique temporal experiences?[3]

A relationship between energy expenditure and heart rate has been uncovered: rapid heart rate implies an intense metabolic rate and an allegretto pace of living (men, in raising their heart rates from 100 to 150 beats per minute doubled their metabolic rates).[4] Abnormal metab-

---

1. Sams, H.V., Aging: the loss of temporal organization, Perspectives in Biology and Medicine, Autumn, 1968, 95-102.
2. Hirsch, H.R., The multistep theory of aging: relation to the forbidden clone theory. Mechanisms of Aging and Development, Vol. 3, 1974, 165-172.
3. Webster, I.W., Aging and the relativity of time, J. Amer. Geriatric Society, Vol. XXIV, No. 7, 1976, 314-6.
4. Morhardt, J.E., S.S. Morhardt, Correlations between heart rate and oxygen consumption in rodents, Am. J. Physiology, Vol. 221, No. 6, 1971, 1580-5.

olism in disease may manifest itself by loss of weight in diabetes and increased skin temperature in fever.[1] In 1908 Rubner showed that the food consumed in the body yielded the same amount of evolved heat as the equivalent amount burned in vitro (outside the body). Atwater and Benedict constructed a whole-body oxygen chamber in which men could live and work for days at a time, where their oxygen consumption and hence metabolic rates could be continuously monitored. Subjects with diabetes, anemia and malaria were the objects of an inquiry into the effects of these conditions on metabolism. In 1894 the impact of food, age, and sex, goiter and myxedema on BMR were studied. Basal metabolic measurements were of assistance in the diagnosis and treatment of diseases of the thyroid gland, though it was recognized that the BMR recorded was not necessarily the lowest metabolic values obtainable; prolonged undernutrition as well as sleep produce even lower readings. For normal men of the same size and age we can expect a 10 percent variation in BMR determinations. There will be a few between 10 and 15 percent of the average. Within the same individual we also find differences: perhaps 5 percent higher in cold versus hot weather and dependent upon the time of day. Children in the vital phase of life have high BMR values (twice adult levels) as their bodies develop and change rapidly. There is a peak in early life, one to 10 years of age, after which the BMR gradually declines. Per unit weight, embryos exhibit the greatest BMR, apparently a reflection of the work of differentiation. In so-called cold-blooded animals (which assume the temperature of the surroundings) metabolism increases rapidly with the air or water temperature of their environment. Warm-blooded animals protected by thick fur or a heavy layer of subcutaneous fat do not show the same instability for environment variations of 20 to 30°C. We regulate heat loss from our bodies by evaporation, radiation, and conduction and convection. Should we find ourselves in a hot, humid ambience, these modes of heat transfer may be

---

1. DuBois, E.F., Basal metabolsim in health and disease, Lea & Febiger, Philadelphia, 1927.

insufficient to prevent hyperthermia which triggers an aberrant rise in the metabolic rate. When things get too cold, we shiver and thereby raise the metabolic rate. Dogs exposed to cold are able to shift water from their blood to the skin and subcutaneous tissue. In the lowered pressures of space capsules, BMR values drop by 5 to 20 percent. Persons in the tropics average a 6 percent lower than standard BMR. In general, Japanese and Chinese show slightly lower basal metabolic rates than Americans or Europeans. Caucasians going to the tropics experience a gradual decrease in body heat production. Vegetarians or those on low protein diets have lower metabolic rates than non-vegetarians with high protein consumption. During sleep there is a marked fall in metabolism associated with a drop in pulse rate.

It's clear enough that life as we know it cannot be maintained even in cold-blooded animals without the production of heat. The amount of heat evolution is naturally greater in warm-blooded creatures whose body temperatures are almost always above that of the surrounding air. One quarter of the heat generated is lost through the evaporation of water from the skin and lungs and consequently must be accounted for in calculating basal metabolic rates. Heart action generates about 4 percent of our metabolic heat; breathing movements about 10 percent; kidney metabolism may be 5 percent; other organ functions total 25 percent. Three-quarters of the heat produced under BMR conditions is derived from chemical reactions in the resting tissue, all controlled by the thyroid. Remove the thyroid and you diminish the BMR by 40 percent. At birth the liver and the thyroid are larger than for adults, perhaps explaining why the young can establish relatively high basal metabolic rates. Children consume greater quantities of food in proportion to their body weight. Are the consequences an accelerated rate of living and a foreshortened longevity? The higher metabolism of children may be caused by a growth factor and the onset of puberty. Some typical average BMR values, per kilogram of body weight are: horses, 11.3; pigs, 19.1; man, 32.1; dogs, 51.5; rabbits, 75.1; geese, 66.7; fowl,

71.0; mice, 212.0. We should exercise a note of caution in interpreting these numbers; there are no ages reported. As we know by now, BMR values diminish with age after peaking in the early youthful stage of life and so we cannot readily compare them, except to glean a rough relationship between BMR and longevity. The mouse is short-lived (highest BMR), the horse is longest-lived (lowest BMR) if we exclude humans who seem to be the exception here. Obese men, heavier than 90 percent of their cohort group or more than 15 percent overweight had basal metabolic rates which were less than the average by 13 to 25 percent, raising a question as to whether their obesity might be caused not so much by overeating but by the inability of their bodies to assimilate and "burn" the food efficiently. Conversely, thinner persons (lighter than 90 percent of the rest or more than 15 percent underweight) showed BMR values greater than average by 5 to 7 percent, indicating perhaps a more rapid rate of living.

With fever or hyperthyroidism the patient may become undernourished though consuming a normal diet simply by virtue of the elevated metabolic processes occurring. Underfeeding or starvation then leads to a restoration of the proper metabolic rate. Consider the interesting case of A. Levanzine, aged 40, who fasted for 31 days during which time he received nothing but water. His body temperature showed surprisingly little change from normal; during the last 10 days of the fast his temperature was only 0.2 to 0.4°C lower than initially. The average sleeping pulse rate which was 64 to 76 dropped to 55 beats per minute on the tenth day and to 49 on the seventeenth day whereupon it rose to and stayed at 55 for the remainder of the fast. The loss in body weight during the early part of the fast was in part due to the loss of water; liver and muscle glycogen was consumed. When the glycogen stores became low on the third day, fat and protein metabolism became significant, protein utilization engendering about 15 percent of the total calories. (The amino acids derived from the protein catabolism in one organ can be used for the regeneration of another, as in the case of the salmon during the spawning season who fasts for many days, yet in spite of great muscular activity can still deposit large amounts of new tissue in the reproductive glands.) In fasting our body is selective: the muscles and glandular organs suffer most of the fat and protein loss, the skeleton and nervous system least. (What would happen to rapidly growing tumors in a starving subject?) The basal metabolic rate dropped markedly during Levanzine's fast, diminished by 30 percent in 21 days. When the glycogen stores were reduced to a point where carbohydrate metabolism fell below the critical minimum we began to see the metabolism of fats, i.e. the secretion of ketone bodies in the urine, a diseased condition called ketosis, similar to diabetes. Some students with normal diets of 3200-3600 calories per day were placed on a restricted diet of 1400 calories per day for three weeks without reducing their mental or physical activities. As a consequence of this regimen, BMR values dropped 20 percent, pulse rate was down, systolic and diastolic pressures were distinctly lowered.

One of our chief carbohydrate foodstuffs is starch, a polysaccharide. When ingested, our saliva and pancreatic juices convert the starch to glucose, with the chemical formula $C_6H_{12}O_6$. As such it is absorbed through the intestinal wall into the blood and eventually oxidized (reacts with oxygen) in the cells to form carbon dioxide, water and heat. Oxidation—or combustion—liberates heat as will any other fuel. In burning glucose, the volume of carbon dioxide produced is theoretically, exactly equal to the volume of oxygen consumed and we say that the respiratory quotient, R.Q., the ratio of carbon dioxide to oxygen is equal to 1.0 for carbohydrate oxidation. Fats furnish about a third of our calories normally but a much larger proportion in starvation and diabetes. The fats enter the intestines where they are broken down into their constituent fatty acids by enzymes and the bile secretion from the pancreas, finally wending their way to the blood. In the blood the suspension of fatty acids causes a slight milkiness of the plasma which persists for 8 to 14 hours after the fat-containing meal. The metabolism or oxidation of fats with oxygen yields carbon dioxide and water and heat; the respiratory quotient for this is around 0.7, the amount of carbon dioxide liberated for each unit of oxygen consumed. Fats furnished more heat compared to carbohydrate metabolism (in the ratio of 9.3 to 4.1). Proteins, constituting about 19 percent of the human body, are composed of large numbers of amino acids. In the stomach protein foods are rapidly deracinated by hydrochloric acid and pepsin into smaller constituents. When in the intestines, further severed linkages yield the amino acids which are absorbed into the blood stream. This is the material for tissue replacement. Amino acids also are oxidized to furnish energy and heat as do carbohydrates and fats. Protein metabolism releases sulfur and nitrogen compounds which are eliminated through the kidneys. Nitrogen excretion in the urine is used as an index of protein metabolism. Infectious diseases associated with toxemia, cancer and other wasting illnesses are accompanied by the destruction of protein (nitrogen excretion exceeds nitrogen food intake). Metabolism of protein with oxygen yields the usual carbon dioxide, water and heat and a respiration quotient of around 0.8. Diabetics have BMR values higher than average, on the order of 20 percent above average, attributed to extraordinarily high protein metabolism. Enlargement of the thyroid and growths on it can raise the BMR by 30 percent. Removal of these benign growths (adenomas) or treatment with iodine (for goiter) can improve things. Graves' or Basedow's disease is derived from an abnormal secretion of thyroxine from an enlarged thyroid, resulting in hyperthyroidism: high BMR values, manifestations of nervousness, vomiting and diarrhea. Iodine administration will usually cause a remission in symptoms. On the other hand, a seriously diminished level of thyroxine secretion yields a disease called myxedema (BMR down 40 percent) which is reversible with doses of thyroxine. Malignancies of the thyroid usually will elevate the BMR. Normal basal metabolic rates generally are subsumed within a 15 percent range (above or below) of the standard values. Very severe cases of goiter show an increase in

BMR of 75 percent above average; mild cases less than 50 percent. Anemia, leukemia and polycythemia simulate hyperthyroidism: BMR up 11 to 90 percent. Diseases characterized by BMR values elevated beyond 11 percent of normal are: hypertension, endocarditis; myocarditis; pericarditis, malignancies in general, acromegaly; splenic and pernicious anemia, lymphatic and myelogenous leukemia. Diseases yielding less than 11 percent of normal BMR values are: epilepsy; some malignancies; dysphagia, hypopituitarianism. Considering only the thyroid, diseases producing greater than 11 percent BMR readings were goiter and adenomas while the below 11 percent category included myxedema, hypothyroidism and thyroiditis. Cretinism is characterized by a BMR 22 to 35 percent below normal.

Pulse rate is a rough approximator of basal metabolism. Pulse rate multiplied by pulse pressure seems to be even more accurate, an empirical formula successful within 10 percent in predicting BMR. Without any thyroid secretion of thyroxine patients will exhibit BMR values 40 percent below normal. Thyroxine given to normal men caused the expected increase in BMR and produced symptoms of Graves' disease. Removing adrenal glands from dogs and cats produced a depression in BMR and body temperature. (Adrenaline can raise the respiratory quotient and the BMR by 10 to 20 percent.) BMR values in leukemia may be as high as in incidences of Graves' disease, 20 percent above average, even 40 to 80 percent in acute cases. Polycythemia, a disease accompanied by a great increase in the number of red cells and hemoglobin shows a BMR elevation of 10 to 42 percent (when fever is at its highest). Patients with malaria raise their heat production during the chill. With fever there may be a 10 to 40 percent rise in the basal metabolic rate; generally BMR follows body temperature and hence the degree of the fever: a 13 percent rise in heat production for each degree centigrade augmentation in body temperature. In lobar pneumonia, values of the BMR 20 to 50 percent above normal seem to be usual. Caffeine raises the BMR, on the order of 10 to 20 percent. Body temperature in a baby falls precipitously immediately after birth.[1] Full term infants at birth are able to adjust their BMR values upwards about 10 percent in response to cold; oxygen consumption drops when the environmental temperature is lowered below 32 to 36°C. Hibernating animals maintain their body within a few degrees of the ambient temperature.[2]

Whether performing mechanical work or not, just staying alive requires energy. Cells do work in transporting solutes across cell membranes.[3] Some, especially muscle cells do mechanical work, much of which is internal such as in pumping blood. Heat is generated within the body while we sleep and of course during our waking hours. Ten to 30 percent of the energy expenditure during mechanical work is applied externally; the remainder evolves as heat. A man asleep may operate at a level as low as 1 kilocalorie per minute (77 watts per minute). When doing sustained hard work he may generate 15 kilocalories per minute (1155 watts per minute). Some organs of our body such as the brain oxidize fuel at a high and steady rate throughout the day; the liver and skeletal muscle are more variable, the skin more indolent. Since skeletal muscle is about 40 percent of the body mass, a change in its heat production becomes a dominant factor when counting the BMR. The heart and kidneys have similar metabolic rates; the brain and muscle are about 60 percent higher.[4] For every liter of oxygen consumed, 4.7 to 5.0 kilocalories of heat is released.[5] When we do muscular work there is an immediate energy release from the consumption of ATP

---

1. Hill, J.R., K.A. Rahimtulla, Heat balance and the metabolic rate of newborn babies in relation to environmental temperature, J. Physiol, Vol. 180, 1965, 239-265.
2. Henshaw, R.E., Thermoregulation during hibernation, J.Theoret. Biol., Vol. 20, 1968, 79-90.
3. Webb, P., Work heat and oxygen cost, in Bioastronautics data book, Second edition, NASA SP-3006, 1973.
4. Altman, P.L., D.S. Dittmer, editors, Metabolism, Bethesda, Maryland, Federation of Amer. Soc. of Exp. Biology, 1968.
5. Maxfield, M.E., P. Smith, Abbreviated methods for the measurement of oxygen consumption in work physiology, Human Factors, Vol. 9, 1967, 587-594.

(adenosine triphosphate) and phosphocreatinine, followed later by a replenishment from carbohydrate (glucose and glycogen) fuel stores. Some of the energy may be applied to do external work, the rest to maintain our internal muscle tone, the excess rejected as heat. Work causes a rise in muscle temperature, the heat conducted to the skin and elsewhere via blood flow. This heat loss from the body must balance that which is generated internally to maintain isothermal conditions. The heart muscle accelerates its energy and heat production with exercise; the brain does not. Sleeping of course results in the lowest heat generation; very light, seated activities such as writing and typing may yield BMR values 50 to 100 percent above the minimum sleep levels. Light efforts, playing musical instruments, ironing, slow walking, show three times the sleep levels; moderate efforts, slow swimming, cycling, baseball pitching and tennis give 5 to 6 times the lowest sleep levels; heavy activities, strenuous swimming, rapid bicycle riding, chopping wood, rapid stairs climbing and soccer generate 8 to 9 times sleep level; very heavy work, very rapid cycling, serious basketball playing, very rapid stairs climbing and wrestling yield heat production rates 13 to 16 times the sleeping levels. Over a sustained period swimming the breast stroke at 3 miles per hour seems to be the most strenuous activity reported: 97 times more heat production than sleeping while the butterfly stroke at 3 miles per hour is next at 75 times the sleep value.[1] Maximum work capacity as measured by oxygen consumption reaches its peak in the late teens and twenties, then declines slowly as we age. The effect of physical conditioning programs on untrained but otherwise healthy men is to increase their maximum breathing capacity by 10 to 20 percent.[2] Maximal efforts lasting perhaps one to two minutes is anaerobic work, that is, your muscles get energy by splitting phosphate bonds and glycogen as contrasted

---

1. Altman, P.L., J.F. Gibson, C.C. Wang, Handbook of respiration, WADC TR 58-352 Aero Medical Laboratory, Wright Air Development Center, Wright Patterson AFB, Ohio, August, 1958.
2. Astrand, P.O., K. Rodahl, Textbook of work physiology, New York, McGraw Hill, 1970.

with aerobic work which involves oxidation of carbohydrates and fats and can be sustained for ten minutes or more. After heavy anaerobic work, some of the oxygen present is used to oxidize one of the end products of the anaerobic process, lactic acid.

For each of us there is an internal temperature at which we are comfortable, give or take about 0.3°C. At internal temperatures above this set point, vasodilation and active sweating occur; below this set point, vasoconstriction and increased metabolism due to shivering commences. Under steady-state conditions, the metabolic energy is dissipated as work accomplished and heat rejected to the atmosphere. Under proper resting conditions defined as the basal state, most of the metabolic energy is lost to the surrounding air and this is what we measure as the basal metabolic rate (BMR). Heat loss due to respiration varies directly with the metabolic rate and is influenced by carbon dioxide and water vapor in the air. Heat loss from the lungs approximates 10 percent of the metabolic heat.[1] The basal state is a standardized set of experimental conditions agreed upon as being as close as possible to a physiologically and psychologically neutral milieu in which to measure the BMR. The subject must be in a post-absorptive stage of digestion to avoid any of the effects of food ingestion and digestion on metabolic activity (12 to 15 hours after the last meal), should have slept well, should not have done anything strenuous before the test and reclined for 30 minutes before it, must be comfortable and calm to minimize the level of activity of the sympathetic nervous system which secretes norepinephrine, and be in a thermally neutral environment, 62 to 87°F (which minimizes the effects of increased muscle tone (shivering or sweating). In 1678 it was observed that a shrew mouse would die of asphyxiation in a sealed vessel containing a burning candle. In 1770 measurements of the composition of man's inspired and expired air showed changes in oxygen, carbon dioxide and water vapor. A little later heat evolution from

---

1. Hardy, J.D., editor, The physiological problems in space exploration, Springfield, Ill, C.C. Thomas, 1954.

living guinea pigs was quantified. By the early 1800's we knew that some sort of combustion of foodstuffs was occurring inside animals. Around 1840 we understood this was oxidation of carbohydrates, fats and protein. The respiration quotient was measured in 1850 and found to vary from 0.62 to 1.04, depending on the foods consumed and the health of the animal. A whole-body calorimeter was constructed in the late 1870's which could maintain a man and monitor his oxygen consumption for long periods of time. Basic work on heats of combustion of various foodstuffs was accomplished in 1894. Human calorimetry became more sophisticated and accurate by 1897.

Metabolism comes from the Greek word meaning the act or process of change; it is defined in terms of the intrinsic energy utilized by living systems, which comes basically from our food supply. Not all of this potential energy is available; what energy we finally capture is generally stored in the form of adenosine triphosphate (ATP) or creatine phosphate (CP). Both contain the high energy phosphate bond. In living, ATP is transmogrified to ADP (adenosine diphosphate) as one phosphate bond is broken to release its bound energy. The level of ATP in the body remains relatively constant, assisted by CP, acting as a reserve source of phosphate. When ATP is being metabolized (oxidized) to ADP—as in a muscle or nerve cell when active—the creatine phosphate (CP) donates its phosphate group to ADP to rejuvenate the ATP. CP becomes creatine. In measuring the BMR, under the prescribed stable resting conditions, all of the food energy is converted to evolved heat, the BMR heat. There are thousands of chemical reactions in the various biochemical pathways we call the living process, but we categorize them generally in terms of the oxidation of carbohydrates, fats (or lipids) and protein:

$C_6H_{12}O_6 + 6O_2 \rightarrow 6\ CO_2 + 6H_2O$ carbohydrate (glucose)
respiration quotient = $\frac{6}{6}$ = 1.00

$$2C_{51}H_{38}O_6 + 146\ O_2 \rightarrow 102\ CO_2 + 98H_2O \quad \text{fats (tripalmitin)}$$

$$\text{respiration quotient} = \frac{102}{146} = 0.703$$

$$2C_6H_{13}O_2N + 15O_2 \rightarrow 11CO_2 + 11H_2O + CO(NH_2)$$
$$\text{urea}$$

protein (amino acid leuceine)
respiration quotient = $\frac{11}{15}$ = 0.734

These reactions are exothermic; they proceed with the evolution of heat. We find in general that carbohydrates liberate 4.1 kilocalories for each gram oxidized; fats, 9.3 kilocalories per gram; protein, 5.6 kilocalories per gram. Heat production is an indication of our vitality or rate of living. In humans this metabolic rate is about 60 to 70 kilocalories per hour; during violent activity it may achieve a burst of 1000 to 2000 kilocalories in an hour or 200 to 300 kilocalories per hour over a sustained period. Men have basal metabolic rates (BMR) 5 to 7 percent above women's values. It seems Orientals have lower BMR readings than Caucasians; Indians (Eskimos) are higher. Two hormones secreted by the thyroid gland, thyroxine and triiodothyronine affect the BMR dramatically: thyroxine by its absence may cause a 50 percent decrease or in excess can change this to a 100 percent increase. The male sex hormone, testosterone, can hike the BMR by 10 to 15 percent; curiously, the female sex hormone, progesterone, seems to have a negligible effect on the BMR. The somatotrophic (growth) hormone of the pituitary raises the BMR 15 to 20 percent. Epinephrine and norepinephrine secreted by the sympathetic nervous system and the adrenal glands can kite the BMR 60 to 100 percent for short periods. If your BMR is between -15 percent and + 20 percent of average, it is considered normal. Between -30 percent and -60 percent we begin to suspect hypothyroidism and a possible lack of thyroxine in the cells. BMR values, + 50 percent to + 75 percent, are inferred to be signs of hyperthyroidism, an overactive thyroid, too much thyroxine leaking into the cells. Caffeine increases the BMR, 2, 4-dinitrophenol in small quantities ups the BMR by a stupendous 1000 percent. Cancer, leukemia, polycythemia, anemia, cardiac failure, hypertension, Cushing's disease and infections or febrile conditions can cause elevated BMR values. Diseases of the adrenal and pituitary glands proscribe undersecretion (Addison's disease). Eating tends to raise the metabolic rate; it takes 2 to 5 hours for the carbohydrates effect to subside, 7 to 9 hours for fats, 10 to 12 hours for protein. Undernourishment or fasting drops the BMR by 20 to 30 percent. Metabolic heat generation is increased by a departure in either direction from our thermal comfort zone of 26 to 27°C. Persons in highly emotional states may experience basal metabolic rates 20 to 30 percent above normal; sleep on the other hand is characterized by BMR values 10 to 15 percent below average.

The basal metabolic rate, measured under very specific experimental conditions, depends ultimately on two major factors: the inherent velocity of the chemical reactions in the cells and the amount of thyroxine secreted by the thyroid which activates them. A stressful environment, such as an atmospheric pressure half of normal or with less oxygen content than usual necessitates adjustments; respiration and blood circulation as well as red cell and hemoglobin production are affected[1]: in rats we see an initial lowering of the rectal temperature followed in a few days by an adaptation, whence the temperature returns to normal. (In old animals restoration is not complete.) Young rats experience diminished body weight and inhibited growth when exposed to low barometric pressures or low concentrations of oxygen in an otherwise normal environment. It is not known what causes the drop in body temperature initially but it is probably related to a diminished heat production, a particular problem for old animals. This inability to adapt is an immanent, early sign of aging. On the other hand, mice with skin cancers, exposed to hyperbaric hydrogen atmospheres (2.5 percent oxygen, 97.5 percent hydrogen, 8

---

1. Verzar, F., E. Fluckiger, Adaptation to low atmospheric pressure, Symposia and Abstracts, Internat. Assoc. of Gerontology, Third Congress, 1954, 263.

atmospheres pressure, for two weeks) showed a marked regression of the tumors.[1] Here we seem to have two factors involved: (1) an ambience poor in oxygen, which should be helpful in minimizing the free radical reactions believed to be deleterious to our longevity and immune systems and hence a dolorous influence on cancer growth (hydrogen in itself may be a free radical neutralizer) and (2) high pressure, an intensifier of whatever other effects are expected. It is not yet clear from these results whether the observations are permanent, whether there are as yet undetected harmful effects derived from the hydrogen environment. We are caught in a cruel bind in that oxygen which supports our lives is also a toxic substance by virtue of its ability to produce the free radicals so damaging to our living processes.[2] The margin of safety is so narrow: we can be killed by exposure to 5 to 10 times the normal concentration of oxygen in the air. Some bacteria are unable to survive in the presence of any oxygen. Observed similarities between the lethality of oxygen and ionizing radiation led in 1954 to the theory that free radicals were the root cause of oxygen toxicity. In general we have these possibilities: (1) oxygen plus an electron goes to O_2^- (the superoxide free radical); (2) oxygen plus electrons plus hydrogen ions gives hydrogen peroxide; (3) oxygen plus electrons plus hydrogen ions yields water and O_H (the hydroxyl free radical); (4) oxygen plus electrons plus hydrogen ions becomes water. We have some natural defenses against the various free radicals. One receiving great attention these days is SOD (superoxide dismutase), an enzyme which catalyzes (enhances) the breakdown of the superoxide free radical O_2^- to hydrogen peroxide and subsequently to innocuous water. Numerous spontaneous chemical reactions in the body generate substantial amounts of superoxide free radicals; the basis for oxygen toxicity could reside here. Perhaps the most damaging reaction O_2^- can undergo is that with hydrogen peroxide,

---

1. Dole, M., F.R. Wilson, Hyperbaric hydrogen therapy; a possible treatment for cancer, Science, Vol. 190, Oct. 10, 1975, 152-4.
2. Fridovich, I., Oxygen: boon or bane, American Scientist, Vol. 63, Jan.-Feb., 1975, 54-9.

H_2O_2. One of the products is the hydroxyl free radical, O_H^-, the most potent oxidant known. Capable of attacking virtually any of the organic substances found in cells, it accounts for a large fraction of the biological damage wrought by ionizing radiation. We believe any system which generates the superoxide free radical will soon accumulate hydrogen peroxide which will then react with the continuing flux of superoxide free radicals to generate the hydroxyl free radical. If this is the problem in aging, then the solution is apparent: keep the concentrations of the superoxide free radical and hydrogen peroxide as small as possible, accomplished by SOD enzymes that scavenge these free radicals. Also we want to reduce the hydrogen peroxide to water and hence break the chain reaction. Superoxide dismutase (SOD) is present in the copper-containing and zinc-containing forms in bovine red cells. Manganese-containing SOD is found in some bacteria such as E. Coli and also in chicken livers. A fourth type, iron-containing, is likewise obtained from E. Coli. Copper and zinc SOD have been isolated in humans, cows, chickens, spinach, yeast and bread mold. Aerobic organisms (who can live in the presence of oxygen and utilize it in the biochemical reactions) have significant levels of SOD in their cells whereas anaerobic creatures (unable to survive in an oxygen environment) have none. The adaptation of rats to an abnormal atmosphere of 85 and 100 percent oxygen is associated with an increase in the amounts of SOD in their lungs. The antibiotic, streptonigrin, is much more toxic to the bacterium, E. Coli, in the presence of oxygen than in its absence. Streptonigrin is here a superoxide generator. If SOD is indeed the biological defense against the superoxide free radical, the E. Coli containing elevated levels of SOD should be resistant to the aerobic lethality of streptonigrin, which is the case.

The study of heat generation in living systems gained its first firm footing as a result of the experimental work of the French investigators in the eighteenth and nineteenth centuries, Lavoisier, Laplace, Benard, D'Arsonnal,

Regnault and others.[1] A healthy person does not survive with an internal body temperature beyond the normal range of 36°C to 38°C although during strenuous work and in febrile disease we may tolerate for short periods temperature as high as 40°C to 41°C. Denaturation (breakdown) of vital cellular protein occurs so rapidly at 44°C to 46°C that pain is evoked and tissue death comes after a few hours. We may also be able to tolerate hypothermia (low temperatures) for brief durations with body temperatures as low as 27°C to 29°C. An average-sized man in the sitting position produces approximately 70 kilocalories each hour; nude subjects in an environment at 3°C initiate shivering in less than 3 minutes, raising the metabolic rate and warming the person. We tend to begin shivering at 12°C. Exercise will raise the metabolic rate (rectal temperatures reflect this). In a comfortable, thermally neutral environment, women demonstrate lower heat production than do men. In uncomfortably warm surroundings women are able to dilate their blood vessels more rapidly than men and therefore had less sweating. In cold exposures, women indicated much greater discomfort, perhaps due to their lower metabolic rates. Old people become increasingly erratic in their responses to their environment. Given an upset in temperature, diet, physical activity or emotional stress, the powers of adjustment of the old are weaker than for the young systems. Mostly we describe this problem in terms of a diminished feedback response or faulty homeostasis, but the actual reasons, on the microscopic level, are still not known. Why is it that old age robs us of the vitality and control of our faculties? If we age and die because of the depletion of some inborn quantity of energy, then we need to find a way of unwinding the life clock more slowly. We need to find a way of decreasing the rate of living, improving the efficiency of living. Can we account for the wear and tear of dashing for trains and buses, and the myriad of other heart-stressing, dizzying

---

1. Hardis, J.D., J.A.J. Stolwyk, A.P. Gagge, Man, Chapter 5, in Comparative physiology of thermoregulation, Vol. II, Mammals, G.C. Wirtow, editor, Academic Press, 1971.

activities which exhaust our bodies and minds? Can we invent a better measure of age, based not on years but on some physiologic parameter? Some are old at twenty, others are young at fifty.

A relationship between longevity and metabolic rate was first suggested by Rubner and Pearl[1]: the total basal metabolic expenditure from maturity to death in several animal species was about 200 kilocalories per gram of body weight. Fruit flies at elevated environmental temperatures demonstrated shorter longevity than control groups. (If we are "blessed" with a fixed energy potential, higher temperatures increase the rate of consumption of this energy and we die sooner.) Or is it the product of longevity potential and heart rate which is the true invariant, regardless of ambient conditions or sex of the species? A few experiments show the effects of exercise on lifespan; for rats on revolving drums, those that exercised lived longer than the controls. This seemed true for young rats but not for older ones. And what does that mean for us? During sleep, mammals lower both their body temperature (0.5°F to 1°F) and their BMR (10 to 20 percent). For many animals, multiplying the averaged daily BMR by the maximum longevity potential is a constant, running to 200,000 kilocalories for each gram of body weight.[2] As the size of the species shrinks (shrews and small mice) the BMR per unit weight becomes inordinately gross, suggesting that perhaps there is a lower limit to multicellular mammalian dimensions beyond which the BMR is impossibly large (the higher the metabolic rate, the shorter the lifespan)[3], on the order of 2.5 grams for the shrew.

What we call metabolism is the sum total of the various chemical processes of muscle contraction, nerve impulse conduction, glandular secretions, growth, tissue

---

1. Sohal, R.S., Metabolic rate and lifespan, in Interdisciplinary topics in gerontology, Vol. 9, 1976, 25-40.
2. Cutler, R.G., Nature of aging and life maintenance processes, in Interdisciplinary topics in gerontology, Vol. 9, 1976, 83-133.
3. Tracy, C.R., Minimum size of mammalian homeotherms: role of environment, Science, Vol. 198, Dec. 9, 1977, 1034-5.

repair and reproduction, etc. We oxidize carbon and hydrogen stored in the foods ingested—carbohydrates, fats and protein—to yield carbon dioxide and water and concomitantly, energy. A measure of the rate of living, or our vitality is the basal metabolic rate (BMR), obtained by analyzing the oxygen consumed (the indirect method) or the heat evolved (the direct method). The BMR, obtained under properly specified resting conditions, accounts for the heat evolved from the heart, liver, brain, kidneys and muscles. Its magnitude is a function of physical size, age and sex. A growing child, relative to its size, has a considerably higher BMR than the adult because the child spends a great deal of energy in synthesizing new tissue. On the other end of the age scale, the metabolic cost of living gradually decreases with advancing age. The brain, liver and muscles utilize the greatest percentage of oxygen (and generate therefore the most metabolic heat), followed by the heart, adipose (fatty) tissue and kidneys.[1] The major energy requirement in basic maintenance functions is for nervous control, then heart work, protein resynthesis (muscles, liver, intestines), respiration (muscle work), kidney function (sodium transport) and triglyceride resynthesis (in the fatty tissue and the liver). About 10 percent of the basal energy expenditure goes for resynthesis of protein. If our body temperature could be lowered safely by 10°C, the metabolic rate might be reduced by a factor of 2.5. At dangerously high temperatures, the destruction of tissue is far more rapid than can be repaired by metabolic activity. Exercise is perhaps the most powerful stimulus for the metabolic rate: in muscle contraction a tremendous quantity of ATP is changed to ADP. During very strenuous exercise lasting only a moment the metabolic rate can soar to 40 times normal. When the sympathetic nervous system is stimulated, norepinephrine is released directly into the tissue by the sympathetic nerve endings. This hormone and epinephrine are released into the blood by the adrenal

---

1. Baldwin, R.L., N.E. Smith, Molecular control of energy metabolism, in J.D. Sink, editor, The control of metabolism, Penn., Penn State University Press, 1974.

medullae. The two hormones exert a direct effect on all cells, raising their metabolic rates and encouraging the breakdown of glycogen into glucose. Intense stimulation can drive the metabolic rate up by 160 percent, lasting but for a few minutes after the temporal signals cease. The thyroid hormone, thyroxine, works on cells also, like norepinephrine, except that thyroxine requires several days to take effect, but then continues acting for as long as 4 to 8 weeks after its release from the thyroid. Thyroxine can increase the metabolic rate up to 200 percent of normal; a complete lack of thyroxine cuts it down by 50 percent. Insulin from the pancreas, growth hormone from the pituitary, testosterone from the testes and adrenal cortical hormones raise the BMR 5 to 15 percent. All are affected by temperature, of course: 10 percent for each degree centigrade change; with high fever our metabolic rate may be twice normal. After a meal, the BMR usually is elevated and remains so for 2 to 10 hours: fats and carbohydrates, 4 to 15 percent; protein, 30 to 60 percent. Basal metabolic rates are obtained under "basal" conditions: the subject has not exercised during the last 30 to 60 minutes, the subject is at mental rest (the sympathetic nervous system is not overactive); comfortable ambient temperatures, no food intake within the last 12 hours; normal body temperature. In the basal state most of the factors affecting the metabolic processes are controlled. Thus we are in actuality measuring (1) the rate of the chemical reactions in the body (our vitality or rate of living) and (2) the amount and efficiency of thyroxine action on our cells. Though all tissue produces heat, those incorporating rapid chemical reactions produce the predominant amounts. In this resting state the liver, heart, brain and most of the endocrine glands are the major heat generators, causing their temperatures to be a degree or so higher than the rest of the body. In this basal state the heat evolved from skeletal muscle function is not great but because half of the entire mass of the body is muscle, the summed total reaches 30 percent of the entire BMR. During severe exercise muscle heat generation may achieve 20 times that of the rest. A nude body may lose 60 percent of its heat by radiation to the walls of the room, 22 percent by evaporation, 15 percent by heat conduction to the air in the room and 3 percent by conduction to whatever we are sitting on; core body temperature may vary by 1°F when exposed to extremely cold or hot weather. Extreme emotions can do the same; exhaustive exercise produces a 5°F to 6°F change. Located in the hypothalamus are neurons that respond directly to and control temperature by sensing the thermal condition of the blood flowing into the preoptic region. Sensing cold, we respond with vasoconstriction (the blood vessels of the skin constrict, decreasing the flow of warm blood from the internal organs to the skin) thereby diminishing the loss from these heat producing organs. The temperature of the skin falls towards the surrounding value. The heat promoting center raises our degree of wakefulness and increases muscle tone (thereby stimulating muscle heat production). These taut muscles soon begin to oscillate and we have shivering. Exposed to cold for several weeks—as at the beginning of winter—our thyroid augments its output of thyroxine, where over a period of weeks there may be a 20 to 40 percent bulge in heat production. On the other hand, in high temperature environments, everything is reversed and instead of vasoconstriction, the blood vessels dilate, allowing the skin to become very warm so that heat can be lost rapidly. Muscle tone is eased, thyroxine production drops as does heat generation. Sweating and panting ensues. The hypothalamus acts as a thermostat, maintaining our internal body temperature within half a degree of average. Fever causes an aberration. The most frequent cause of fever is bacterial and viral infection such as occurs in pneumonia, typhoid, tuberculosis, diphtheria, measles, yellow fever, mumps, poliomyelitis, etc. Collateral effects are obtained from severe heart attack, x-rays and other radiation exposures. Fever is usually caused by abnormal protein release into our body fluids during the disease process (raising the hypothalamus temperature set-point). When this happens, there is a call for more heat—as will our furnace after we've raised the thermostat setting—and the body responds by doing those things which raise its temperature, including vasoconstriction, higher metabolic rates driven by norepinephrine secretion and finally shivering. The skin is cold. In time we reach the thermostat setting and the chills disappear but our temperature remains regulated at the higher setting until something occurs to interrupt the disease process, whereupon the thermostat setting is lowered to normal and the heat losing mechanisms come into play, particularly vasodilation and sweating. Our skin now becomes warm and we begin to sweat (a sign our temperature is beginning to fall). Fever and the concomitant elevated body temperature may be beneficial as a mechanism for combating infection since many bacterial and viral agents do not survive as well at high temperatures. Or is it that the major benefits are derived from speedier chemical reactions which accelerate cell repair mechanisms? However, above 108°F to 110°F our temperature regulatory mechanisms seem unable to restore the original conditions; cellular metabolism becomes too great, control is lost and we "burn up". The neurons of the brain suffer permanent damage even though the patient may recover. Inversely, should body temperature become pathologically depressed, heat regulation again becomes impaired: sluggish chemical reactions and heat metabolism. Death usually comes when we reach about 75°F. [1,2,3,4]

BMR values for 8,614 normal persons showed that 77 percent fell within 10 percent (above or below) of average and 90 percent were within 15 percent. It is customary to consider 15 percent as the normal variation

---

1. Benzinger, T.H., Heat regulation, homeostasis of the central temperature in man, Physiol. Review, Vol. 49, 1969, 671.
2. Chauffee, R.R.J., J.C. Roberts, Temperature acclimitization in birds and mammals, Ann. Rev. Physiology, Vol. 33, 1971, 155.
3. Anon, Adaptation to environment, in Handbook of physiology, Baltimore, Williams & Wilkins, 1965, Section IV.
4. Snell, E.S.F. Atkins, The mechanisms of fever, in The biological basis of medicine, Bittar, E.E., N. Bittar, editors, NY, 1958, Vol. I, 397, Academic Press.

from the accepted standards.[1,2] Body temperatures which deviate from normal can affect BMR by 13 percent for each degree rise.[3] After a meal exclusively of protein, the BMR may increase 20 percent. Compared to the United States, females in India were found to be about 17 percent below average. Chinese women in the U.S. were 10 percent lower. Uncertainties redound from the variations in climate, altitude and drug involvement. Caffeine, epinephrine and thyroxine charge the BMR. Thiouricil blocks thyroxine production, dropping the BMR. The ultimate heat production we seem capable of developing is about 4 times the BMR value. (For rodents this factor is 7.) In rats this maximum metabolic rate can be maintained for only 3 to 20 minutes.[4] Shivering and muscle tone are important sources of heat production. In most homeotherms shivering can increase the metabolic rate 2 to 3 times (perhaps even 5 times) the BMR. Since no mechanical work is done during shivering, all the energy released by muscular contractions appears as heat. Nevertheless shivering is not a very economical process of heat control because the increased blood flow to the exterior surfaces (from the shivering) simply accelerates the heat loss; only 48 percent of the extra heat generated by shivering is retained.

Small mammals running at their limits on a treadmill extended their metabolic rates to 4 to 8 times the BMR; for humans, simply moving your arms raises the metabolic rate to twice the basal metabolic rate; running, 3 to 10 times. Trained athletes at peak performance can generate a 20-fold higher heat production.[5] Our skeletal muscles can generate 50 percent

---

1. Brobeck, J.R., Energy exchange, in medical physiology, V. Mountcastle, editor, Saunders, Philadelphia, 1978.
2. Boothby, W.M., J. Berkson, W.A. Plummer, The variability of basal metabolism, Ann. Intern. Med., Vol. II, 1937, 1014.
3. DuBois, E.F., Basal metabolism in health and disease, 3rd Edition, Philadelphia, Lea & Febiger, 1936.
4. Jansky, L., Heat production in body temperature, Lomax, P., E. Schonbaum, editors, Marcel Dekker, New York, 1979.
5. Salton, B., P.O. Astrand, Maximal oxygen uptake in athletes, J. Applied Physiology, Vol. 23, 1967, 353-8.

of the total heat produced.[1] Epinephrine, which can increase the metabolic rate 30 to 100 percent, has been detected in the urine during nonshivering exercises in concentrations 500 percent above standard. Epinephrine may come into play when norepinephrine by itself is unable to meet our energetic requirements.[2] Thyroxine, though capable of stimulating metabolism does have a time delay associated with its efficiency, apparently on the order of several days. It is suspected that thyroxine enables norepinephrine and epinephrine to do their work.[3] Sleeping generally requires about 0.172 kilocalories energy per kilogram of body weight for each 10 minutes and is the lowest metabolic rate we normally record during a 24 hour day. In order of increasing metabolic rates we have: standing, 0.206; driving a car, 0.438; walking downstairs, 0.976 and walking upstairs, 2.540.[4] Most of the energy generated by our chemical reactions appears immediately as heat; only a small fraction is used for work. It is customary to divide biological work into two general categories: (1) external work, i.e., movement of objects by contracting skeletal muscles and (2) internal work, all the other biological activity. All internal work is ultimately transformed into heat except during periods of growth. And if the subject is lying at rest (during basal metabolism measurements) there is no external work and essentially all the biological activity manifests itself as heat generation or the BMR. Internal work may be: heart blood pumping (which reappears as frictional heat); secretions of hydrochloric acid in the stomach and sodium bicarbonate in the pancreas (which yields heat when the hydrogen and bicarbonate ions react in the small intestines); the ATP

---

1. Jansky, L., J.S. Hart, Cardiac output and organ blood flow in warm and cold acclimated rats exposed to cold, Can. J. Physiol. Pharmacol, Vol. 46, 1968, 653-9.
2. Jansky, L., Nonshivering thermogenesis and its thermoregulatory significance, Biol. Rev., Vol. 48, 1973, 85-132.
3. Jansky, L., Heat production, in body temperature, Loman, P., E. Schonbaum, editors, Marcel Dekker, N.Y., 1979, 89.
4. Brobeck, J.R., Energy balance and food intake, in Medical physiology, 13th edition, V.B. Mountcastle, editor, Sanders, Phila., 1979, 1253.

chemical reactions. The total energy liberated when body nutrients are broken down (catabolized) may be transformed into body heat, appear as external work or be stored (during periods of growth). Changes in muscle activity greatly affect BMR values which may partly explain the drop during sleep and even the rise we see during the emotional stresses capable of unleashing unconscious, roiling muscular activity (epinephrine and thyroxine may be released). Intravenous injection of epinephrine can elevate our heat production 30 percent, probably due to the stimulation of glycogen and triglyceride breakdown. Thyroxine affects most body tissue except the brain; excessive amounts leads to hyperthyroidism where our metabolic demands are so dramatic compared to our inadequate diet that we begin to consume body protein and fat stores, leading to loss of weight, weakened muscles and bones, vitamin deficiencies, increased heart rate and an intolerance to warm environments. A man of 150 pounds, awake and lying still requires 77 kilocalories per hour for survival, while walking at 2.6 miles per hour he generates 200 kilocalories per hour. Other values are: sexual intercourse, 280; jogging at 5.3 miles per hour, 570; working at maximul output, 1,440.

In 1908 Rubner hypothesized that there was a limiting lifetime energy expenditure potential for mammals and put the figure at 200 kilocalories per gram of body weight.[1] The connection of lifespan to metabolic rate and lifespan to brain size, body weight and temperature have been expressed. You can separate metabolism into (1) the BMR component and (2) the activity increment and look for specific correlations with longevity. However, birds with body temperatures as much as 5°C higher than their corresponding mammals of equal size and metabolic rate nevertheless exhibit life expectancies considerably greater than the mammals.[2] (So metabolic

---

1. Sacher, G.A., P.H. Duffy, Genetic relation of lifespan to metabolic rate for inbred mouse strains and their hybrids, Fed. Proceedings, Vol. 38, No. 2, Feb., 1979, 184-8.
2. Flower, S.S., Contribution to our knowledge of the duration of life in vertebrate animals, V. Mammals, Proc. Soc. of London, 1931, 145-234.

rate alone may not be the arbiter of longevity.) Environmental poisons affect us, as do the misformed products of our chemistry, illnesses, accidents and nutrition.

Divide the metabolic rate by body temperature. This ratio is a general measure of our entropy production, of which more will be said later, but for now let's allow that entropy is related to the randomness or disorder within us. We live—and die—by descending from a highly ordered system to an increasingly disordered state, towards the ultimate disorder, death. Entropy increases as disorder increases. At a given age—comparing two persons—the one with a higher rate of entropy production is living at a faster pace and less efficiently and will die sooner (if we are allowed to slide towards senile death). As we age, the rate of entropy production is curtailed, but nevertheless continues relentlessly. Thus entropy production may be the tocsin to mark our life's progress: rapid when we are young; slow when we are old. Sacher[1] imputes significance to the product of BMR and the square of lifespan, suggesting this becomes a universal constant for all of us. Others find the rate and amount of DNA repair correlates well with lifespan for shrews and mice to elephants and man. (Human beings live about twice as long as gorillas and chimpanzees and have DNA repair rates about twice as great.)

Our life's processes run their course with some sort of measure of order. The second law of thermodynamics, or the law of entropy, states that every natural phenomenon proceeding of its own volition leads finally to an increase in disorder. The evolution of living systems is sometimes explained by so-called random mistakes which happen now and then. Isolated systems tend towards equilibrium with their surroundings where they achieve maximum disorder and entropy. So we ask, What is life? Is it orderly?[2] The tendency of living organisms is to organize their surroundings but this does not imply a violation of the second law of thermodynamics. The missing link in

---

1. Sacher, G.A., Longevity and aging in vertebrate evolution, Bioscience, Vol. 28, No. 8, Aug., 1978, 497-501.
2. Riedle, R., Order in living organisms, Wiley, New York, 1979, 4.

the argument is the recognition that we are dealing with open systems where energy and matter can invade our system. It is the summed disorder or entropy produced within us, on and around us which must always be increasing. So if the birth of a baby seems to produce a highly organized (more ordered) state, or the painting of the Mona Lisa from bits and dabs of paints, we must not lose sight of the rest of the Universe which becomes a little more disorganized as a result. And the total, the circumscribed system and that beyond adds up to a higher entropy level than before.

From the field of information theory there is a way of measuring our degree of surprise in the outcome of an event; we call this "information content" and connect it to probabilities, but in an obverse way. The less something is possible or the more ways there are to do it (the greater the degree of uncertainty), the more information content there is. In the simplest case, that of tossing a coin, the probability of the next event being tails is one in two, or 1/2. The reciprocal or inverse of this is 2 and we say the information content is 2 bits (derived from the digital computer yes-no decision). The formula relating information content in bits and probability is $I = \log_2 R$, or $I = \log_2 \frac{1}{P}$ which says that information, I, is equal to the logarithm of $\frac{1}{P}$ where P is the probability fraction of an event, R is the number of possibilities and the logarithm is based on the number 2. Another way of looking at this is $2^I = \frac{1}{P}$; the number 2 is raised to the Ith power. Suppose for example we have a roulette wheel with 32 equally probable positions. Then for each chance or event, the odds are $P = \frac{1}{32}$ or one chance in 32 possibilities of winning. In the formula given here, $2^I = \frac{1}{1/32} = 32$, or I = 5 bits and we can say that we must make five decisions in order to select one successful event out of 32. However, if the occurrence of an event can be predicted with certainty, then all surprise disappears, P = 1 and I = 0 (the information content has disappeared). In every chain of events, the information content reaches a maximum when all events are set by accident. From these ideas can be derived a concept of entropy. For example, when we melt a solid, its entropy increases by the heat added to melt it, divided by the melting temperature. The material, in being transformed from an ordered, firm structure to a more uncertain fluid has increased its disorder content. The disorder is that of the motion of atoms being mixed at random instead of being neatly separated in the solid. We recognize the natural tendency of things to approach a chaotic state unless we impose outside forces. Every closed physical system changes as its entropy increases, from a less probable to a more probable condition, by $S = k \cdot \log P$, where k is the Boltzmann constant, S is entropy and P, probability. Or $I = k \log R$, where $R = \frac{1}{P}$ is the number of possibilities and we now measure information, I, in the same units as entropy. In our roulette wheel example, with $P = \frac{1}{32}$, $R = 32$ which are the number of possibilities. Information turns out to be exactly that which is known in thermodynamics as entropy, for it becomes a question of possibilities and freedom of choice. The greater the uncertainty initially, the greater is R (the possibilities) and the larger will be the amount of information required to make the selection. Consider the sequence of tossing a coin with outcomes 0 (heads) and 1 (tails). Therefore a sequence of symbols (0011010...) carries specific information. Tossing a coin yields events 1 and 0, two different possible events, $R = 2$. In playing dice, one die has six different outcomes (1,2,3,4,5,6) and $R = 6$. The result of tossing a coin or throwing a die is interpreted as receiving one message out of R outcomes. The greater R, the greater the uncertainty before the message is received and the larger will be the amount of information after the message is received. Initially we have no information and I = 0). A binary system has only two symbols or letters (the head and tail of a coin, yes or no answers to a question) translated into the numbers 0 and 1. Forming words or sequences, of length n in these binary systems gives $R = 2^n$ different possible events (n = 1, head-tail, R = 2; n = 2, head-tail, R = 4, etc.). We previously defined information, as $I = \log_2 R$ or $2^I = R$, so that when $R = 8$, $I = 3$ bits.

Information may be considered a measure of an event's lack of predictability or the dearth of knowledge. It is identical with the number of decisions which are required to explain a phenomenon, or to describe it, or to establish it. Such information increases with the range of the numbers (of symbols or possibilities) and with the disorder or entropy. Order may be formulated from the content of governing laws, multiplied by the number of instances when the laws apply. Is there another phenomenon we know whose order begins to approach that of the life process? Life requires a flow of energy from a source to a sink and work must be performed continuously, as we tend always towards the equilibrium of death. Order could correspond to the difference between the free energy of living and death, the tension between the storing of energy and its decay as we drift towards the most random possible configuration. When we bring a cold object in contact with a hot one, heat is exchanged so that eventually both bodies acquire the same temperature. The system has become thermally homogeneous. The reverse process, however, is never observed in nature. Thus the direction of a natural process is unique. A drop of ink in water will spread until finally the color is distributed uniformly. The spontaneous assembly of ink from its solution to an ink drop is never observed. Consider a moving car whose engine is suddenly shut off. Eventually the motion ceases as the kinetic (motion) energy is abased by frictional forces, converting the kinetic energy into heat (warming the wheels, engine parts, etc.). The organized, ordered energy has been transformed into a disordered form. Entropy, the measurer of the degree of disorder can chart the course of these changes as its value increases. On the other hand we can manipulate a system from beyond its borders, and improve its degree of order—and hence lower its entropy. For example, water vapor in the form of steam at high temperatures is composed of freely moving molecules, seemingly in random motion. Should we lower the temperature, eventually a liquid drop of water will be formed in which the molecules now possess some sort of regular distance between themselves. Their motions are much more circumscribed. At still lesser temperatures, at the freezing point, liquid water becomes ice crystals in which the molecules are arranged in a fixed order. The same molecules are involved in each phase change but we observed some obvious changes and we say the entropy of the ice crystals is less than that of the steam. Order has been imposed. The cost of doing this is derived from the heat exchanged and the work required to move the heat. The entropy content of the outside world in which the intervening forces were at work has been raised, this increment more than balancing the loss of entropy of the steam to water to ice transformation. Thus the entropy of the universe, system and surroundings has been increased and there is a bit more disorder abounding. Biological processes do not achieve order by the lowering of temperatures but by maintaining a flux of energy and matter. Energy is fed into the system in the form of chemical energy (food) which eventually results in ordered phenomena (growth, protein synthesis, locomotion, etc.). Out of chaotic states we are able to marshall the forces for self-organization.

The property of self-organization is a fundamental feature of living systems. It is reflected in evolution as well as in the development of limbs and other functional appendiges. But in getting from here to there the self-organizing systems, particularly living organisms, don't necessarily travel in direct, linear steps, but rather in oscillatory fits and starts.[1] Biological order results from chemical reactions and mass and heat transfer, driving us away from steady, unchanging equilibrium. It is clearly recognized that biological systems are irreversibly organized (they seem to grow and evolve) which is one of the most striking and intriguing aspects of natural phenomena: complex systems, involving large numbers of strongly interacting elements, can form and maintain patterns of order. From the most elemental levels of chemical reactions to the macroscopic development of multicellular beings such as we are, or even for societal

---

1. Hess, B., Oscillations. A property of organized systems, in Frontiers in physicochemical biology, B. Pullman, editor, Academic Press, New York, 1978, 409-419.

systems, concepts such as regulation, information and communications play prominent roles. What are the driving forces inducing such coherent behavior? Is it the permanent or transient differences in concentrations of matter and energy? We are in reality alluding to the thermodynamics of irreversible processes, pioneered by Ilya Prigogine[1,2,3] who proposed that the transition from an ordered, biological or chemical state to another ordered state requires a critical distance from equilibrium. As we stray further and further from our equilibrium, there is a point reached when our stable state becomes unstable and we then evolve towards a new regime, a new ordered state; the transition is governed by stability criteria based on excess entropy production (the dissipation introduced by the disturbances driving us from our equilibrium). Systems with the potential for making such transitions are generally non-linear, that is, they tend to have complex relationships describing their behavior: enzyme behavior in our bodies; chlorophyll-induced plant growth; some fluid motions; cell membranes. Fluctuations are an essential aspect of evolution in living systems driven from equilibrium; eventually the decisive fluctuation is produced, the chaotic evolutionary phase is ended and a new stable state is attained. Under these nonequilibrium circumstances, entropy production arises from the internal, irreversible processes (this always tends to increase) and from the entropy exchange with the surroundings (which may be positive or negative). A negative entropy flow from the surroundings of such magnitude as to overwhelm the internal, ever positive entropy is the fundamental thermodynamic prerequisite for self-organization.[4,5] For systems not too far from equilibrium there are always stable states characterized by a minimum level of entropy production.[6]

1. Prigogine, I., Etude thermodynamique des processes irreversible, Desoer, Liege, 1947.
2. Glansdorf, P., I. Prigogine, Thermodynamic theory of structure, stability and fluctuation, Wiley-Interscience, New York, 1971.
3. Nicolis, G., I. Prigogine, Self-Organization in nonequilibrium systems, Wiley, New York, 1977.
4. Meixner, J., Ann. Phys., Vol. 43, 1943, 244.
5. Onsager, L., Phys. Rev., Vol. 38, 1931, 2265.
6. Prigogine, I., Bull. Acad. Roy. Belg., Vol. 31, 1945, 600.

Living systems, continuously exchanging energy and matter beget the instabilities which lead to self-organization. Cells can live only if they are fed their chemical diets which enter by diffusion through their membranes. Within the cells, the mitochondria require oxygen, carbon dioxide or light for the biochemical reactions. The cells are open systems, subjected to various transport processes across their membranes, displacing the metabolic pathways from their equilibrium. Which brings us back to information and its increase or decrease as we roam from one state to another. You will recall that information was a uniquely defined measure of probability, a specification of how many yes-no decisions one needs on average in order to achieve a definite result within a given number of alternatives. Hence information relates to complexity. In everyday speech, the concept of information is associated with the content and meaning of an item of news. To inform means to supply someone with knowledge or information. Can the meaning of an item of news be made objective and absolute? Consider the deciphering of a piece of news: the news specialist decodes it from the properties of the language, that is, from the frequency of use of certain linguistic symbols, from the probability of their sequence, from the word lengths, the rules of syntax, etc. Thus it is possible to establish objectively, some predictions of the sense of the news, a meaning to it. What happens in the brain of the news receiver is subjective, dependent on previous history. The system, news and receiver, are an inseparable unit. Information is dependent on certain initial and boundary conditions and is self-organizational in that the brain of the news receiver provides the forces to form it into a coherent pattern of recognition.[1] Then is the self-organization of information an accidental, historically unique confluence of events, or is there some recondite regularity at work? Consider the snowflake, a structure of exceedingly diverse detail,

---

1. Eigen, M. How does information originate? Principles of biological self-organization, in For Ilya Prigogine, S.A. Rice, editor, Wiley, New York, 1979.

containing on average about 10^{18} water molecules 10,000,000,000,000,000). How are we to code a machine to describe the orientation of all these molecules? And this is but one aspect of the problem which confronts us as we attempt to uncover the genetic coding of one of the simplest of living entities, the genetic material of a colibacterium, transmitted from generation to generation by the giant DNA molecule (represented by about 4 million symbols in a linear chain, each symbol using elements of a 4-letter alphabet). Such sentences would have the dimensions of a book of 1000 printed pages; the sequences determining the unique macroscopic characteristics of this bacterium, its ability to metabolize certain substances for energy, self-maintenance and reproduction. There are $10^{2,000,000}$ alternative sequences (10 followed by two million zeroes), a complexity so great that we have practically no chance of achieving by coincidence the correct sequence. This property, to select the proper code and information on the microscopic level we begin to call life. It would seem the life process must fulfill these conditions: (1) The system must possess a metabolism which can build each individual species from energy-rich matter and eliminate energy-deficient products. Metabolism is thus a conversion of free energy, a continuous compensation for the entropy and disorder generated by the irreversible chemical reactions. In this way, the system is blocked from tending inexorably towards an equilibrium state[1]; (2) the system must be self-reproducing. Mutations which may appear because of miscopying can be a source of new information; the system learns from its mistakes.

There has always been a strong connection between living systems and thermodynamics, particularly in the work of Rubner who demonstrated the validity of energy balances in biology and in his study of the metabolism of microorganisms. We recognize today that living matter devolves according to the thermodynamics of irreversible processes, death being the end result of living. We are

---

1. Schrodinger, E., What is Life? Cambridge University Press, New York, 1944.

entropy (disorder) generators; the second law of thermodynamics says, among other things, that life is accompanied by dissipation (heat production). Our living systems are open systems; we add food and air (mass and energy) to our bodies through our boundaries (mouth and skin). There is entropy exchange in breathing as well as that which is generated inside of us. The chemistry of life is irreversible (we can never be the same as before), we proceed with increasing loss and disorder and entropy content. We can measure this entropy production by determining the heat evolved: this dissipation heat, arising from the chemical reactions in us, develops from the degradation of the energy contained in the food we consume. Metabolic reactions, the work of diffusion, osmosis, electrical and mechanical exertions are accompanied by dissipation heat production.[1] One gram of human body weight releases 10,000 times more heat than 1 gram of the sun[2] which gives some indication of the intensity of the life process. A running man releases the same amount of heat per pound weight as does a big ocean liner, the tiny fruit fly while in flight generates heat equivalent to a car riding at the highest speeds, when calculated on an equivalent weight basis; a bacterium is in the same class as a jet airplane.

Thermodynamics and information theory and the extent of order in living systems: they represent a connection that may now be obvious. Some believe the amount of information accumulated in the course of development and growth must drastically increase; others disagree.[3,4] The living system, as an open system, may approach not only equilibrium, but also the stationary state, the difference being that in the latter, the inherent processes occurring across boundaries continue,

---

1. Zotin, A.I. The second law, negentropy, thermodynamics of linear irreversible processes, in Thermodynamics of biological processes, Lamprecht, I., A.I. Zotin, editors, Walter de Gruyter, Berlin, 1978, 21.
2. Calvet, E., H. Prat, Microcalorimetrie, application physico chemiques et biologiques, Masson, Paris, 1956.
3. Brillouin, L., Entropy and growth of an organism, Ann N.Y. Acad, Sci., Vol. 63, 1955, 454-5.
4. Raven, C.P., Oogenesis, Pergammon Press, New York, 1961.

but at a constant rate whereas in equilibrium, things cease to happen. For example, if I have a tank half-filled with water and allow more water to enter at a rate equal to that which is leaving, the tank has achieved a stationary state. No changes are observed in the water level, even though water comes in and exits. On the other hand, should the tank be filled to capacity with hot water and sealed at inlet and outlet and allowed to sit for a long time in an air conditioned room of fixed temperature, we would find that eventually the tank would lose its excess heat and assume the temperature of the room. Thereafter no further changes in tank temperature can be observed and we say the tank has come to equilibrium with its surroundings. In the stationary state entropy production becomes constant and minimal, that is, it is the lowest it can be under the circumstances. In other words, the creation of disorder, while continuing, is at its low ebb. In our approach to senile death, the living system begins to divine the stationary state; our vitality is at a low ebb, our rate of living tends towards a minimum, which may be zero or some critical level below which we lack the energy to maintain the life force.

Living organisms, open and exchanging mass and energy, evolve from life to death by dying a little every day. If you believe the wear and tear (rate of living) theory of aging, we may have within us a certain total entropy potential. Prigogine and Wiame[1] and Prigogine[2,3] applied the principles of the thermodynamics of irreversible processes to the phenomena of development, growth and aging; they assumed living is a process of continuous approach to the final stationary state, accompanied by a steady decline in entropy production (or vitality or rate of living). The stationary state (death) is characterized by a minimum and constant rate of entropy production; we are born, develop, grow and age in a continuous manner, the

---

1. Prigogine, I., J.M. Wiami, Biologie et thermodynamique des phenomenes irreversibles, Experimetia, Vol 2, 1946, 451-3
2. Prigogine, I., Etude thermodynamic des phenomenes irreversibles, Liegen, Desoer, 1947.
3. Prigogine, I., Introduction to thermodynamics of irreversible processes, 3rd edition, Wiley, New York, 1967.

benchmarks being our rate of entropy or disorder accumulation, which can be related to our heat generation and respiration.[1] Data on heat evolution and respiration for animals and humans are available and show the proper trends.[2,3] Animals and humans in the basal state of rest under proper BMR measuring conditions (constant temperature, heart rate, pulse pressure, respiration, etc.) show a minimal level of heat evolution and seem unchanging.

But aren't we in actuality evolving, changing with time but in the short time frame of our observation, it merely seems that we are unchanging. Like it or not we are launched on the parlous journey to the final stationary state and there is no turning back. There may be deviations along the way, brought on by external forces (environmental effects such as air pollution, radiation, etc.) or internal forces (disease or stress) which may induce new norms such as hormonal changes, thyroid dysfunction, etc.).[4]

Immediately after fertilization there is a marked increase in respiration (and heat production) in many animal eggs[5,6]: dramatic in the first minutes after fertilization, less so later. In newborn mice the rise in respiration takes place in 3 to 4 days, attains a maximum 10 to 12 days later and then slowly diminishes.[7] Regulation of body temperature is usually established within 10 days. We behave similarly (the larger the animals, the

---

1. Zotin, A.I., V.A. Grudnitsky, Ratio between the heat production and respiration during animal growth, Ontogenesis, Vol. 1, 1970, 437-444 (Russian).
2. Zotin, A.I., Thermodynamical approach to the problems of development, growth and aging, Moscow, Nauka, 1974 (Russian).
3. Zotin, A.I., Thermodynamic aspects of developmental biology, Basel, Karger, (1972).
4. Ozernyuk, N.D., A.I. Zotin, Y.G. Yurowitzky, Deviation of the living system from the stationary state during oogenesis, Wilhelm Roux Arch, Vol. 172, 1973, 66-74.
5. Rothschild, L., Fertilization, London, Methuen, 1956.
6. Monroy, A., Chemistry and physiology of fertilization, New York, Holt, Rinehart, and Winston, 1965.
7. Walker, M.G., Heat production of the albino mouse during growth, Experimentia, Vol. 23, 1967, 541.

lower are the levels on a unit weight basis).[1] BMR and respiration values in various species of animals have always shown the characteristic decrease after the initial spurt. The white rat, in aging from one to 18 months showed the following decreases in oxygen consumption: muscles, 61 percent; brain, 18 percent; testes, 43 percent; skin, 85 percent; cartilage, 75 percent; kidneys, 19 percent; overall, 57 percent.[2] As we approach senile death in old age, we become progressively weaker and helpless before stresses, unable to overcome them; they now become killing stresses and so we die, not of monumental upsets but because of an inability to restore our former state. Is there a critical level of heat or entropy production below which it is impossible for the living system to support life (our vitality is simply insufficient to maintain the tension of life)? It may not be necessary that life's forces ebb away to nothing and then we die.

Fish continue to grow during the entire lifespan and therefore growth and aging are difficult to differentiate. Mammals and birds are more interesting in this respect since here growth proceeds only in the first third or half of the lifespan. Insects also reach terminal sizes; human growth stops approximately at the age of 20 to 25 years; after this age the BMR diminishes at 3 to 7 percent per decade[3], even in the last stages of aging. But do we achieve that final stationary state where heat production actually reaches a minimum? Zotin and Zotina[4] say we ineluctably move towards such a final stationary state, a condition synonymous with natural death and suggest we

---

1. Zotin, A.I., R.S. Zotina, Experimental basis for qualitative phenomenological theory of development, in Thermodynamics of biological processes, Lamprecht, I., A.I. Zotin, editors, Walter de Gruyter, Berlin, 1978, 61.
2. Nagorny, A.V., V.N. Nikitin, I.N. Bulankin, Problems in aging and longevity, Moscow, State Publ. House Med. Literature, 1963 (Russian).
3. Kise, Y., T. Ochi, Basal metabolism of old people, J. Lab. Clin. Med., Vol. 19, 1934, 1073-9.
4. Zotin, A.I., R.S. Zotina, Experimental basis for qualitative phenomenological theory of development, in Thermodynamics of biological processes, Lamprecht, I., A.I. Zotin, Editors, Walter de Gruyter, Berlin, 1978, 152.

can study embryo development, growth and aging through entropy analysis: the decrease in embryo respiration during its development may relate to the aging process. The mitochondria within the nucleus of our cells, the energizers, increase in concentation in the rat brain between 3 to 33 days after birth, concomitantly with ascending respiration in the brain tissue.[1] And then the brain experiences a loss of mitochondria. In the human liver, we lose them quickly after age 60 and of course simultaneously see a fall in oxygen respiration. Each new organism begins its development from a maximum level of heat or entropy production.[2] This ability to start from zero, achieve a maximum and then decline is of utmost interest not only in the study of normal aging, but also as we explore regeneration of organs and tissue, wound healing and malignant growth. Do we rake in the energy or entropy credits, achieve a maximum and then, sufficiently activated, enter the pathway of development and growth?[3] The amputation of the posterior part of an earthworm at segment 60 is followed by an increase in oxygen respiration, attributed to the wound infliction. Soon respiration diminishes, followed by a new wave of respiration stimulation which is related to the regeneration of the earthworm segments.This reflexive respiration increase is found not only in the earthworm, but also in mammals and other animals during regeneration of the liver.[4,5] Maximum metabolic rates are attained somewhere in the middle of the regeneration stage and then gradually return to normal. Do we need an energy

---

1. Samson, F.E., W.M. Balfour, R.J. Jacobs, Mitochondrial changes in developing rat brain, Amer. J. Physiol., Vol. 199, 1960, 696.
2. Samson, F.E., W.M. Balfour, R.J. Jacobs, Mitochondrial changes in developing rat brain, Amer. J. Physiol, vol. 199, 1960, 696.
3. Zotin, A.I., R.S. Zotina, Experimental basis for qualitative phenomenological theory of development, in Thermodynamics of Biological processes, Lamprecht, I., A.I. Zotin, editors, Walter de Gruyter, Berlin, 1978, 1954.
4. Needham, A.E., Regeneration and growth, in Fundamental aspects of normal and malignant growth, Amsterdam, Elsevier, 1960, 588-663.
5. Sidorova, V.F., Z.A. Ryabinia, E.M. Leikina, Liver regeneration in mammals, Moscow, Medizina, 1966 (Russian).

expenditure of unusual intensity to drive the cells towards repair or regeneration? Some research suggests this, the work having been done on axolotls of various ages[1], which showed approximately the same critical level of oxygen respiration. In some dissembled way cancer cells represent rejuvenated cells, with high rates of metabolic heat (entropy) production, but their rejuvenation happens to prevent the resuming of the normal process of aging; cancer cells attain a high metabolic rate and maintain it. With malignancy there may be an augmented concentration of mitochondria in the cells.[2]

For living systems at rest, with the chemical reactions proceeding relatively slowly, all of the internal heat generation evolved becomes equivalent to entropy production and is measured by the heat lost to the environment.[3] The living system with age passes from a less probable state to a more probable one: the most probable state being death. In the course of development, growth and aging, each event is accompanied by its characteristic heat evolution.[4] Thus the continuous recording of heat evolution ought to detect fluctuations of the vital functions in subcellular biochemical systems as well as in isolated organs or in the whole organism.[5]

---

1. Vladimirova, I.G., I.S. Nikolskaja, Age changes in respiration intensity in the course of tail regeneration in axolotl, Ontogenesis, Vol. 2, 1971, 502-6 (Russian).
2. Vilenchik, M.M., Changes in cytoplasmic DNA during cell malignization, Adv. Mod. Biol., Vol. 75, 1973, 388-405 (Russian).
3. Zotin, A.I., R.S. Zotina, V.A. Konoplev, Theoretical basis for a qualitative phenomenological theory of development, in Thermodynamics of biological processes, Lamprecht, I., A.I. Zotin, editors, Walter de Gruyter, Berlin, 1978, 85-98.
4. Presnov, E.V., Strengthened evolution criterion in development biology, in Thermodynamics of biological processes, Lamprecht, I., A.I. Zotin, editors, Walter de Gruyter, Berlin, 1978.
5. Schaarschmidt, B., I. Lamprecht, Heat production in life processes, in Thermodynamics of biological processes, I. Lamprecht, A.I. Zotin, editors, Walter de Gruyter, Berlin, 1978.

These measurements have been made in the past.[1-7] Drinking water can provoke a sweating response and heat generation. Patients with different kinds of anemia showed elevated rates of heat production. If the heat cannot escape from the environment which has captured it, as in microbial accumulations in hay, wool, manure, and alcoholic fermentation, spontaneous combustion and fires can result. Temperatures as high as 265°C can be found in moist hay.[8] If there is no heat regulation, living systems will die. For humans, special mechanisms have been developed to dissipate the heat: through blood circulation for example. (We maintain a constant temperature independent of the varying environmental temperatures.) Yet in a beehive, a constant temperature is maintained summer and winter by the collective contributions of all the bees in the hive, whose individual heat evolution is variable but controlled to produce the constant ambience. In microorganisms, a large part of the heat generation is due to the cell division process, whereas in higher animals such as humans, the heat originates mainly from muscular contractions and from glandular activities controlled by the nervous system. Bacteria live far from equilibrium and exhibit higher heat production

---

1. Hershey, D., H.H. Wang, A new age-scale for humans, Lexington Books, D.C. Health, Lexington, Mass., 1980.
2. Tiemann, J., Ein respirationkalorimeter zur bestimmung des transformationgrades des der verbrennung in menschin organisms, Elektro-medizin, Vol. 14, 1969, 135-145.
3. Carlson, L.D., N. Honda, T. Sasiki, W.W. Judy, A human calorimeter, Proc. Soc. Exp. Biol. Med., vol. 117, 1964, 327-338.
4. Benzing, T.H., R.G. Huebscher, D. Minard, D. Kitzinger, Human calorimetry by means of the gradient principle, J. Appl. Physiol., Vol. 12, 1958, 1-24.
5. Snellen, J.W., D. Mitchell, M. Busansky, Calorimetric analysis of the effect of drinking saline solution on whole body sweating, Pluger, Arch. des Physiol., Vol. 333, 1972, 124-144.
6. Eldblom, E., Hauttemperaturmessung bei ischias, Klin Wschr, Vol. 14, 1935, 639-41.
   Richter, A., Die stromungkalorimetrie und ihre verwendbarkeit bei der diagnostik peripherer durchblutings-storungen, 1959.
8. Hussain, H.H., Okolgische untersuchungen uber die bedeutung thermophiler mikroorganismen fur die selbsterhitzung von heu, Z. Allg. Mikrobiol., Vol. 13, 1973, 323-34.

(and entropy generation) than we do, on a unit weight basis. Somehow we have learned to moderate our rate of living, perhaps by controlling our body temperature.[1]

The formation of metabolic heat may result in a local increase in temperature and the self-acceleration of the living process itself.[2] The smaller the organism, the higher is its oxygen respiration and heat production, per unit weight. We say: smaller animals are farther from equilibrium (more rapid dissipative processes) than larger ones. This is true in embryonic development. When we are far from equilibrium we are more prone to produce new systems and structures—dissipative structures—driven by the rapid influx of energy into these far from equilibrium, irreversible processes. The metabolic heat ineluctably leads us to these new dissipative structures and is what we call growing up.[3-7] The metabolic heat may be accompanied by thermal, infrared radiation which may be absorbed in the surrounding tissue, energizing the cellular matrix, inducing some sort of cycling pattern to the life process. If this is correct, one can imagine the mitochondria within our cells adventitiously acting as energy oscillators, fixing the energy here, releasing it there, building electrical fields in the membranes, heightening ATP reactivity and causing an activated transport through cellular membranes.

We aim to remain unchanged, as if that were possible. Instead we plod towards evolution: an ascendance from

---

1. Schaarschmidt, B., I. Lamprecht, Heat production in life processes, in Thermodynamics of biological processes, I. Lamprecht, A.I. Zotin, editors, Walter de Gruyter, Berlin, 1978.
2. Zotin, A.I., Dissipative structures, in thermodynamics of biological processes, Lamprecht, I., A.I. Zotin, editors, Walter de Gruyter, Berlin, 1978, 158.
3. Prigogine, I., Structure, dissipation and life, in Theoretical physics and biology, North Holland, 1969, 23-52.
4. Prigogine, I., La thermodynamique de la vie, Recherche, Vol. 3, 1972, 547-62.
5. Nicolis, G., Stability and dissipative structure in open systems far from equilibrium, Adv. Chem. Phys., Vol. 19, 1971, 209-224.
6. Glansdorf, P., I. Prigogine, Thermodynamic theory of structure, stability and fluctuations, London, Wiley, 1971.
7. Prigogine, I., G. Nicolis, Biological order, structure and instabilities, Quart. Rev. Biophys. Vol. 4, 1971, 107-148.

birth to maturity and then the decline—gradual, immutable, unstoppable towards death, the final equilibrium condition. The governing boards of corporations deplore the status quo, for fear that stockholders will interpret this as stagnation. Countries, like corporations, search for an ever-increasing gross national product, eschewing any interest in limiting production. Don't look back, bigger is better. A cessation in the upward spiral is tantamount to senescence; and we all know that civilizations decline and die. Do you prefer to remain close to equilibrium and allow that small perturbations can be handled in a way that returns us to our original state? The living process may operate this way in the short term but in the greater span of time, we are always changing, evolving. So we march from one stable state to the next, each new, differing from the old; but new is not always better. Often there is no choice for us. Is the life of a living system to be seen as a wear and tear process as we wind down or is it a gradual diachronic trip from birth through intermediate states to maturity, senescence and death? For structures such as corporations, it is not readily apparent that they age and die, though some will go bankrupt, which is a form of death. Civilizations die in some way. There have been golden ages of Greece and Rome and perhaps even for the United States. Who can say that the feral forces at work on civilizations are not similar to those which stress a living human system.

There are many avenues open for a changing system. Some change agents force the change, though many of us resist and are comforted by the "olden" days. If the speed limit on a highway is 55 miles per hour and you are law abiding, you might average that speed over the long run yet there will be times when you travel at 60 or 50. You always strive to return to the speed limit, reigned in by an innate morality or the fear of the speeding ticket. The earth in its rotation around the sun traces an orbit which is cyclic and predictable. These two examples illustrate the neutrally stable condition. On the other hand, a poorly designed nuclear reactor, one with improper temperature control generates more and more heat as the nuclear reactions are fed by the ever rising energy levels. (Definitely an unstable condition heading for disaster.) Or perhaps we are tracing the loss of middle-class persons from the inner cities. With the departure of some, the tax bite intensifies for those who remain, schools deteriorate, crime increases and more middle-class persons flee to the suburbs and exurbs. This then exacerbates the initial problem—only now the degree of difficulty has been raised and more flights occur. The trend is unappetizing unless there is outside intervention or the group members themselves alter the pattern. Another example of an unstable condition. A third mode for causing change is typified by the negotiating process between persons or complex organizations, such as in successful bargaining: the system converges to a well-defined end point. Here we have a narrowing of differences and a graceful evolution towards a compromise. Such a system usually is aided by immanent moderating influences which prevent blowups, that is, they negate the uncontrolled growth of stress. It is as if the system were carefully delimited by outside forces. Finally there is the cycle where it is possible to arrive at the desired end by a number of differing paths: a spinning top, no matter what initial rotation is imposed will always end at rest. Death as the ultimate end, is approached by all of us in different ways, but the preordained fey conclusion is the same.

Growth within fixed structures must sooner or later bump against countervailing forces. The dinosauer attained a critical size, beyond which it was impossible to support its immense body weight. This unwieldy girth could have affected dinosauer survivability by limiting its ability to forage for food. Some are more adaptable, able to be transformed to a state in equilibrium with the environment. The cockroach, for example, seems perfectly suited for our present civilization. There are those who say organizations procede to and through various plateaus, resting on each level until displaced by the convergent fluxes of energy, material and information. The human body can be examined anew in this light; we maintain a relatively stable, though changing condition until an illness alters our lives; a corporation operates under known, steady conditions until it merges with another corporation. And so it goes, open systems being driven from one seemingly stable orbit of operations into another. Organizations near equilibrium attempt to meet new pressures for change by damping them and returning to the initial conditions after small, temporary deviations. Some claim the forces of racial integration were like this, where for a while the integrationists' pressures were met by sufficient resistance to prevent change and instead continued the original segregated situation. There was a specious stability in the segregated state but the time frame was not sufficiently long to see the trends. Actually the segregated state was inherently unstable; when the forces for integration became morally irresistible, the system moved to a new nonequilibrium position where we are today. Thus, instead of having a civil war over the issue, society found order through fluctuations. Of course there can be surprises along the way; a system can be driven too far in size and complexity, as some think New York City has been. The high density of its population and the limited network of roads in Manhattan have led to the surprising result that it is often quicker to walk across Manhattan than to drive the same distance in an automobile.

Stability also implies proper negative feedback or return of information to the pressure point. Negative feedback when added to the positive pressure prevents a runaway situation. Should we add positive feedback to a positive pressure point, things begin to add up, increasing the pressure input to the system, yielding a larger output. Part of this positive output is communicated to the pressure point, raising it even more, giving an even higher output, etc. A disaster in the making. Whether considering organizations such as corporations, societal structures such as the welfare system, human living organisms, or the unviverse, what emerges is a general schema for change, a way of traversing the route from one nonequilibrium state to the next: order through fluctuations. This might be called a strategy for revitalization. To get there from here, the system needs to navigate these steps: (1) achieve a plateau; (2) experience stress; (3) endure cultural distortion; (4) plan for revitalization and (5) enter upon a new plateau. Social theories have traditionally been geared to structure, not process and to the ideals of equilibrium and structural stability. The analysis and planning of social organizations now may need to be brought into consonance with the order through fluctuations dicta. Contemporary society is characterized by a rapid dissemination of information. In the past, science and technology were the change agents in the transformation of human-environment relationships, while societal philosophy and techniques provided the negative feedback to stabilize these relationships. A basic tenet of the biological and social universe is the drive towards diversification, heterogeneity and symbiotization (the close relationship of two or more systems). What survives is not necessarily the strongest, but the most symbiotic. We may have been misguided in the past by traditional scientific logic into subscribing to universality, homogenization and competition as not only the rulers of the universe but also the desirable goals for society.

Disorder or randomness is generally related to the definition of entropy; the universe is thought to tend to a uniform distribution of energy and hence towards a state of maximum entropy. This increasing entropy principle is one version of the second law of thermodynamics. Living systems in their developmental stages concentrate energy into highly ordered, tightly organized states and hence accumulate, in a sense, negative entropy. This accumulation of negative entropy is not a violation of the second law of thermodynamics since other contiguous systems increase in entropy and the universe still is inclined to increase its entropy with time (and age), perhaps to a maximum entropy at death. There is not yet a definitive definition of the living state, the best we can do now is describe the major characteristics exhibited by known forms of life. Several traits are obvious: spontaneous movement; irritability; growth and reproduction and the use of nutrients. All living organisms do not show all traits of course; furthermore, some obvious nonliving objects exhibit some of these characteristics, or seem to. Other motifs of life are homeostasis, adaptability, mutability and evolution. Some mammals differing greatly in longevity potential may have equal energy production in their lifetimes: the total metabolic heat given off, measured over the lifetime, seems to be the same (man is the exception with about a fourfold higher figure). This is seen as support for the wear and tear theory of aging (aging depletes the stuff of life, be it energy, enzymes, etc.). Is aging simply a consequence of metabolic activity or entropy production (in highly evolved organisms such as vertebrates this is governed by the size and capacity of the overall information and control system)?[1] Thus we implicitly introduce the concept of the biological clock and suggest that perhaps there is a better way of measuring age, not in seconds, minutes and hours. A lower rate of entropy production permits us to live longer and do more metabolic work. Aging and maturation apparently are related to entropy production of the whole system: aging depends not only on the metabolic work, but also on how well the work is done, in entropy terms. Maximum entropy may correspond to death. We ought to determine entropy production during our lifetimes; comparisons should be enlightening—perhaps we will find a common figure for all of us and all species—and should tell us something about life expectancy.[2] The lifetime heat evolution of various animal species were remarkably similar, of the same order of magnitude.[3]

The human body is a highly improbably and complex system of organs and tissue which involves 60 trillion cells.[4] While the body has a natural mechanism for

---

1. Zeman, K., Entropy and information in science and philosophy, New York, Elsevier, 1975.
2. Hershey, D., Lifespan and factors affecting it, C.C. Thomas, Springfield, Ill., 1974.
3. Hershey, D., Entropy, basal metabolism and life expectancy. Gerontologia, Vol. 7, 1963, 245-50.
4. Guyton, A.C., Textbook of medical physiology, 4th edition, Philadelphia, Saunders, 1971.

restoring cells and combinations of cells to their proper states and functions, the process never results in perfect restoration and alignment of all cells that constitute the body. Thus some imperfections always remain. At first these imperfections are unnoticeable on a macroscopic level; with time, however, more and more cells are not restored to their original configurations and positions. These imperfections gradually accumulate until a critical presence of imperfections is manifested and the entire system collapses; the aging process is always accompanied by the continuous development of errors. Our lifespan depends on factors related to the environment, heredity, life style, nutrition and mental state. One essential feature of living organisms is their ability to capture, transform and store various forms of energy according to specific instructions carried by our genetic material. We need energy to do biological work: our heart pumps blood; intestines absorb foodstuffs; nerve cells supply information. The entropy laws predict energy degradation when doing work, that is, there is always a certain amount of energy which changes into a lower quality and hence becomes less available for further work. It is the law of the universe which applies as far as we know from the smallest atom to the largest galaxy. Entropy increases with the number of cells in our bodies. As we grow beyond some optimal configuration, the disorder level is raised. A system will decay more quickly if insufficient work from its surroundings is applied. The passage of time automatically elevates the entropy of a system unless countervailing forces are applied. As the entropy increases, the degree of random activities follows, yielding extra complexity; our energy becomes less available for doing useful biological work. Aging may be a consequence of this entropy production, triggered by metabolic activity.

Nicolis and Prigogine[1] and Georgescu-Roegen [2,3] are concerned with entropy concepts as applied to evolving structures in chemical, social and economic systems. In biology, order and nonequilibrium phenomena are conjoined; increased complexity leading to increased order is virtually the definition of evolution. In other words, states were derived from nonequilibrium processes, driven towards another form of becoming. Prigogine is interested in the entropy analysis of new structures; one example he cites of a new nonequilibrium form extracted from energy fluctuations is a town, an open system, analogous to the living cell. Georgescu-Roegen says the system of economic thought ignores entropy because of its blind faith in reversibility. He believes that energy, which is consumable, nevertheless is transformed in the direction of increasing entropy, disorder and unavailability and hence something must be lost in the process according to these principles:

(1) there cannot be unlimited substitution of technology and capital for natural resources;
(2) the economic process consists solely of the transformation of low entropy goods into high entropy wastes;
(3) the economic process is irreversible;
(4) it is a myth of the economic profession that resources are properly measured in economic and not entropic terms.

Systems not in equilibrium with their surroundings (but not far from it) evolve until they attain a condition where entropy generation has diminished to a minimum level. Spontaneous fluctuations arising simply regress with time and disappear. Under these circumstances we cannot evolve spontaneously to new and interesting structures. Living systems may be far from equilibrium (there is no gainsaying the relentlessness of the aging

---

1. Nicolis, G., I. Prigogine, Self-organization in nonequilibrium systems, New York, Wiley, 1977.
2. Georgescu-Roegen, N., The entropy law and the economic process, Cambridge, Mass. Harvard University Press, 1971.
3. Georgescu-Roegen, N., Energy and economic myths, New York, Pergammon, 1976.

process) but the rate of change may still reach its nadair in old age: a minimum entropy production which may offer a clue as to the approach of death. So perhaps the nonequilibrium system (which we are) not far from equilibrium—is what we are not. In other words, far from equilibrium we can evolve spontaneously as we age to new structures, sustained by a sufficient flow of energy and matter. Buffeted by pressures and stresses of all kinds, producing fluctuations whose amplitudes become magnified with time, we spontaneously change (we are a self-organized system). This concept is not limited to biological and chemical systems but may be applied to population dynamics, meteorology, economics, the urban existence of a big city (which can survive only as long as food, fuel, information, etc. flow in and wastes flow out) and by extension, corporations and civilizations.[1] We see transitions, the disorganization and disappearance of one structure and the development of another. Near equilibrium we march towards increasing entropy and chaos whereas far from equilibrium the new structures may be highly organized with inestimable complexity. Which path we travel depends on which neighborhood we're in—near or far from equilibrium.

Everything dies eventually, though the lifespans vary. Humans, 85 years of age, have only 10 percent of their cohorts with them, that is, only 10 percent of the original sample is still alive. For the thoroughbred horse, the 10 percent mark is reached at 27, for the laboratory mouse it is 1.5 to 3 years, depending on the strain of mouse.[2] For dogs, survival curves show that the lifespan of large breeds is considerably less than that of smaller breeds. In experiments with rotifers, lowering the temperature of their water environment by 10°C could prolong their longevity about four times its normal expectancy. Diminishing their food intake by one-half extended life three-fold. If I overeat and am constantly

---

1. Hershey, D., H.H. Wang, A new age-scale for humans, Lexington Books, D.C. Heath, Lexington, Mass, 1980.
2. Hershey, D., Lifespan and factors affecting it, C.C. Thomas, Springfield, 1974.

well-fed, will my rate of living be greater than usual? And will I therefore live less than others? (Overfed houseflies are shorter-lived than a control group which is fed normally.) Does it matter how long it takes me to reach full size; and if it does, can I alter my growth rate by control of my diet? (Small apes reach full size at age 3 and live to age 10, while the chimpanzee attains its maximum size at age 11 and lives to age 40.) The ratio of lifespan to age at full size is about 3 to 4 to 1.[1] Slow the growth, lengthen the lifespan? If a woman is fertile, will she outlive others? (For roaches, higher-fertility females have shorter lives than virgin females who lived up to 50 percent longer.) Any lesson to be learned here? If there were something to be learned, would it be worth implementing? If we are crowded together, as we are in many cities, will we have a shorter lifespan? The answer is yes for the drosophila fly. Is it true for us? If I live where the oxygen concentration in the air is low, can that affect my lifespan? Apparently yes for some flies where a pure oxygen environment speeds up the rate of living and shortens life. Does this information on flies apply to humans in their polluted air? The cynical answer is that the oxygen concentration in the polluted air probably will not be a major factor affecting our duration on earth—other pollutants in the air will probably do a better job of killing us.

Radiation exposure cuts our growth and weakens our bodies' reaction to injuries. In exposure experiments on animals, the results indicate that a single radiation dose of 1 roentgen is equivalent in humans to 5 to 10 days of extra age. The radiation also causes increased tumor generation, as if we were older than we really are, when measured by the calendar. Neoplasms, such as leukemia, show up earlier in irradiated mice. Genetic errors are more prevalent after radiation treatment; liver cells of mice show about twice the normal number of chromosome aberrations after a life-shortening dose. With radiation, lesions and degenerative diseases show up in small blood

---

1. Hershey, D., Lifespan and factors affecting it, C. C. Thomas, Springfield, Ill., 1974.

vessels and in the walls of the arterioles. Small arteries are thickened with connective tissue. Fibrous connective tissue is found around the walls of the capillaries. Death from malignant cancer in childhood is about 40 percent higher than normal for children who were x-rayed during the last 3 months of fetal growth than for those who were not. Radiation exposure in a pure oxygen environment is deadlier than in air or pure nitrogen. Radiation shortens life by seemingly accelerating the onset of decrepitude. One dies of old age at a young age. Some diseases simulate the effects of radiation, particularly a disease of children called progeria, a rare disease which transforms the young child into an old person in appearance, with baldness, skin wrinkling and coronary disease. These unfortunate children live only about 8 years. Low doses of x-radiation or γ-radiation are generally not as effective as high-dose rates in shortening the lifespan of animals. This implies that the damage, presumably genetic, is a multihit effect; there is a repair process present which can reverse the damage caused by single hits. Chromosome aberrations in liver cells of mice caused by irradiation (mutations in the somatic cells) are reversible. Life shortening can be induced in adult drosophila flies which are resistant to low doses of radiation by feeding them some amino acids during the larval stage which cause damage similar to radiation damage.

So perhaps a clue to the aging enigma is to be found in the alteration of cells and deoxyribonucleic acid (DNA) by radiation. There are experimental facts which lead in this direction.

1. The lifespan of offspring from irradiated male mice may be shortened almost as much as that of their fathers.
2. The effect of a whole-body radiation dose of 120 roentgens on lifespan is the same whether the radiation exposure is one dose or divided into doses of 20 roentgens.
3. Immature, developing animals are more sensitive to radiation damage than are adult animals.
4. The lifespan of various species is inversely proportional to the mutation rate of the germ cells.

It is generally true that heavier animals or those with large brains tend to live longer. There are also relationships between body weight and metabolic rate (and hence between lifespan and metabolic rate). Those species which have high body weights have low metabolic rates (per gram of weight); thus we may infer in a cautious way that an animal with a low metabolic rate will live longer. Elephants (heavy, with low metabolic rates) live longer than rats (light, with high metabolic rates).

If you raise the very legitimate question about correlating lifespan with brain weight—that it's not the actual weight that counts but the brain weight compared to the total body weight that is significant—you can generate data suggesting that brain weight divided by body weight is a rough predictor of lifespan, allowing for some anomalies such as the results for the crow and parrot.[1] We are smugly reassured, at this stage, to note that humans have the highest relative brain size of all the animals listed. But in our search for more definitive ways of determining the expected lifespan, other available information seems to complicate matters. A mouse heart beats 520 to 570 times per minute. The expected lifespan of a mouse is on the order of 3 years, which yields over the lifetime of a mouse an expected 1 billion heartbeats (approximately). On the other hand, an elephant's heart beats only about 25 times per minute. Its average lifespan might be 80 years. If we do the same type of calculation as we did for the mouse, we see that over the expected lifetime of the elephant, it too will have about 1 billion heartbeats. (In 1908 a theory was presented supporting the finite energy hypothesis. Calculations for total lifetime energy expenditure for horses, cows, guinea pigs, dogs, and cats yielded a figure of 29 to 55 million calories per pound weight of the animal. Humans, the exception, generated 363 million calories per pound.) But it has also been shown that by restricting the diet of immature rats (feeding them nutritious food, but small quantities), it was possible to slow their development, keeping them in a state of

---

1. Hershey, D., Lifespan and factors affecting it, C.C. Thomas, Springfield, Ill., 1974.

immaturity for 766 to 911 days. Longer than usual. Then if the caloric content of the diet was raised, the growth rate was accelerated and the rats matured normally. In the process, however, these special rats had their lives extended about 200 days beyond those who had normal diets. Can life in general be lengthened this way? Perhaps. Did the number of heartbeats for the special rats exceed the 1 billion level expected for the rats with the normal diet? We don't know.

We don't understand much about the simple process of growth; there are some wide ranges of growth characteristics among living things. For example, can you make anything out of the fact that the pygmies of the Ituri Forest in Central Africa average a whopping 8.6 pounds at birth yet only grow to about six times their weight at maturity? They are human beings, as we are, but this growth pattern is not our expected behavior. Some researchers have concentrated on studies of height and weight measurements and other variables as a function of age in an attempt to understand the aging process. There are all sorts of unusual empirical correlation which can be used as predictors of, for example, our final height:

height, inches = 1.88 x length of the thigh bone, inches + 32

which is applicable for grown males. For girls and boys, equations which are good, on the average, for 90 percent of the population are:

girls' height, inches = 2 x height at 18 months, inches + 1/2
boys' height, inches = 2 x height at 2 years, inches + 1/2

We can analyze growth by measuring the height and weight of children. From these experiments it is known that early and late maturing girls have menarche at about the same mean weight, but late maturers are taller at menarche. Two other major events of adolescence, the first spurt in weight gain and the maximum rate of weight gain, also occur at invariant mean weights. These results lead to speculation that a critical body weight may trigger some adolescent events. Or it may be that during maturation the parenchymal cells continue to grow and fill in the space supplied by the capillary bed until the rate of diffusion of one or more limiting nutrients (or the rate of removal of inhibitory products) prevents further growth. We know that the secretion of the estrogen hormone stops female growth. But how? As we grow, we produce more cells; the cells that do not divide get larger. Maggots of the common housefly hatch from eggs with all their cells and generate no more. Their cells simply grow larger and larger with age, accumulate fat, and somehow, when enough fat has been stored, maggot cells cease to grow larger. Having attained this station in life, the maggot stops eating and suddenly a few of its cells begin to divide and differentiate to become wings, legs, eyes, and so on. Human brain cells do not divide, but increase in size and number until we find at age 4 that 90 percent of the growth of the human brain has occurred. On the other hand, human white cells die in 4 days; red cells die in 4 months.

A rough rule of thumb for survival and growth states that lifespan is equal to eight times the age when reproduction is first possible. In some cultures, people eat the reproductive parts of sacrificial animals in an effort to thwart the aging process, hoping for rejuvenation. Injections of the male hormone testosterone can affect the body very dramatically, but this is not true rejuvenation. Brain wave patterns are altered by testosterone injections, as is the chemistry of respiration and nutrition. The red cell count changes and so does muscle tone. But the effects are not lasting and are reversed when the hormone treatment is stopped. In some experiments, cysteine and folic acid were used for rejuvenating effects, but nothing permanent has yet been discovered. Surely we will hear about it when the secret of the fountain of youth is unraveled. Despite the various treatments which are of some temporary help, we continue to age and suffer from skin thinning (glossy appearance of the skin, wrinkling, a decrease in elasticity, and increased pigmentation), hair loss (and graying and coarsening of the texture), eye cataracts (and changes in lens flexibility), muscle loss (through atrophy), joints less flexible (and swollen) and brittle bones.

Some researchers point to the diverse lifespans of various species and say that aging is endogenous and is related to a growth inhibition process, which in turn is related to the time when our fixed adult size is attained. Is it clear to you why the maximum lifespan of the house spider should be 4 days while the longhorn beetle can live to 45 years, the Galapagos tortoise achieves a sensational 177 years of age whereas the swallow lives only 1 year, the rhesus monkey reaches age 29, a chimpanzee can live for 37 years, and the Indian elephant is good for 57 years. Superimposed on these data is the fact that females live longer and have lower basal metabolism rates than males. But are they luckier that they manage to survive for longer periods than their male counterparts? Are they healthy in their old age? Do females live longer because they are subjected to different hormonal influences or is longer life related to the work they do?

The old folks have become an increasing problem for the young as fewer of us die from disease. Though our ultimate, maximum lifespan has not increased very much throughout history, life expectancy has nevertheless increased, as fewer babies die at childbirth and as infants. As diseases are eliminated as the cause of death, life expectancy will increase.

The percentage of the population which is 65 years and older has gradually increased, but note that a larger proportion of the older group is female, since females live longer than males. But women reach their final height sooner than men and they tend to gain weight more steadily into later life than men. What does all this mean?

Much has been written on aging; both scientific and social aspects have been covered. The data are there for those who can avail themselves of a good library.

Many factors which affect the rate of aging of human beings are known. Some are certainly hereditary, others environmental. Senescence probably reflects a complex interaction of hereditary and ecological influences. It is difficult to disentangle the respective roles of nature and nurture in such a highly complex organism as the human being. It is even more difficult to evaluate the action of a particular environmental parameter in a non-experimental situation. Here lies the difference between the approach of the environmental physiologist in the laboratory and the ecologist in the field. The former attempts to keep constant all but one of the environmental variables under study; the latter is faced with a complex of ecological variables, some independent, others more or less obviously correlated. It is little wonder therefore that conclusions drawn from epidemiological surveys have to remain tentative until the experimental gerontologist is able to confirm or disprove them.

The first category of environmental factors includes all the physical and chemical components of the environment, whether natural or due to the unplanned effects of human activity. Important examples are climatic factors (temperature, humidity, and solar radiation), soil and water composition, altitude, various pollutants, and ionizing radiation.[1] Though a good deal of work has been done on their short-term effects, far less is known about their long-term effects.

The second category of environmental factors encompasses all the effects upon humans, whether direct or indirect, of the thousands of living organisms which share the various ecosystems of the world. The living environment exerts its influence upon the human organism mainly through nutrition, pathogenesis, and parasitism.

The paramount importance of nutritional factors upon development and aging processes is well known. Briefly, the great differences in average daily rations between populations arise from (1) the uneven potentialities of artificial ecosystems to produce the kinds of foodstuffs necessary for an optimal functioning of the human organism; (2) the large differences in the efficiency of the various land-use techniques in different

---

1. Comfort, A., Aging: The biology of senescence, New York, Holt, Rinehart & Winston, 1964.

regions and at different levels of technological evolution; and (3) the cultural differences between groups, particularly in the traditional ways of selecting and processing favored foodstuffs. Pathogens and parasites also influence the rate of human development and aging, more particularly in the low-income groups and in tropical countries. This is especially so in tropical Africa, the most disease-ridden area of the world. Until recently human populations were probably more limited by disease than by any other factor. To find the parameters which might measure the lifespan of human beings, we look for information about human physiological adaptability throughout the life sequence. Human adaptive capacity can be thought of as the individual's ability to cope successfully with the stresses of life. Morphological, biochemical, physiological, and psychological processes singly or in combination make this coping response possible. Because their functioning waxes and wanes throughout the individual's life sequence, these processes bring about changes in adaptive capacity.

Eight physiological functions were described by Shock[1] and tabulated by Strehler;[2] namely, maximum breathing capacity, vital capacity, glomerular filtration rate, renal plasma flow, basal metabolic rate, conduction velocity of ulnar nerves, cardiac index, and intracellular water. Values reported were obtained from Bafits[3] and

---

1. Shock, N.W., Some of the facts of aging, Amer. Assoc. Advance Science, Symposium No. 65, Washington, 1960.
2. Strehler, B.L., Origin and comparison of the effects of time and high energy radiations on living systems, Quart, Rev. Biol., Vol. 34, 1959, 117-42.
3. Bafits, H., F. Sargent, Human physiology adaptability through the life sequence, J. Geron., Vol. 32, 1977, 402-480.

others.[1-6] Seven of the eight measurable physiological functions rose from birth to peak or plateau between 1 and 20 years. After age 30 these functions are generally considered excellent indexes of bodily health; all decayed systematically to what might be a critical level—where the curves leveled off (the slope of the curve goes to zero). The ages where the slope is zero are 82, 87, 88, 89, 90, 92 and 95. The arithmetic average was 89. The significance of such critical levels is the question to be explored; it may be the location of the stationary state, the condition of impending death.

Maximal performance of an organ is equivalent to maximal adaptive capacity. Adaptive capacity refers to the ability of the individual to cope with the events of life. It should logically follow that as adaptive capacity decreases the individual will subsequently become unable to withstand deleterious environmental influences and will suffer an increased probability of morbidity and death. In recent years a seasonal variation in mortality in different age groups has been observed. In essence, there is considerable seasonal variation in the death rate in ages 0—4; little seasonality in ages 5—39; and in ages above 40, seasonality again increases. Kutschenreuter[7] postulated that an individual's tolerance of changes in weather decreases with increasing age on reaching age 25. These results clearly lend further support to the concept of physiological function and adaptive capacity

---

1. Brandfonbrener, M.M., Landowne, N.W., Shock, Changes in cardiac output with age, Circulation, Vol. 12, 1955, 557-66.
2. Brillouin, L., Am. Sci., Vol. 37, 1949, 554.
3. Davies, D.F., N.W. Shock, Age changes in glomerular filtration rate, effective renal plasma flow and tubular excretory capacity in adult males, J. Clin. Invest., Vol. 29, 1950, 496-507.
4. Norris, A.H., N.W. Shock, I.H. Wagman, Age changes in the maximum conduction velocity of motor fibers of human ulnar nerves, J. Appl. Physiol., Vol. 5, 1953, 589-93.
5. Norris, A.H., N.W. Shock, M. Landowne, A. Folozone, Pulmonary function studies: age difference in lung volumes and bellows function, Gerontology, Vol. 11, 1956, 379-87.
6. Shock, N.W., M.J. Yiengst, Age changes in basal respiratory measurements and metabolism in males, J. Gerontology, Vol. 10, 1955, 31-40.
7. Kutschenreuter, P.H., Weather does affect mortality, Am. Soc. Heat. and Refrig., Air Cond. Eng. J., Sept. 1960, 39-43.

variability. The younger age group (5—19 years) is able to cope with seasonal variation in weather and does not exhibit seasonality. The very young and older persons cannot cope as well and thus show seasonal trends. This is consistent with the fact that there is poor, incompletely developed temperature control in the very young and impairment of control in older individuals.

It is well known that the age range for maximal athletic performance is in the early 20's for short-distance tasks and 25—30 in endurance events. This is consistent with our profile of adaptive capacity. Simonson[1] studied the effect of age on various types of performance and related physiological functions. He found that maximal oxygen uptake, which is the best reference level for aerobic work capacity, decreased with age. The speed of initial increase in oxygen consumed in work and oxidative recovery were delayed as one aged; the mechanical efficiency remained unchanged or moderately decreased in older age groups. He also found that respiratory efficiency, cardiac stroke volume, muscle strength and endurance (under moderately heavy work) all decreased with age, but endurance in static work remained unchanged with age. Pulse rate recovery was delayed and the speed of repeating movements by small muscles was slightly decreased, while motor coordination in small and larger muscles was unchanged and well maintained. Terris[2] proposed that health could be redefined in functional as well as subjective terms. He urged the development of an epidemiology of health, using the measurement of performance capacity to provide a scientifically valid framework. A well-integrated epidemiology of health must include the concept of adaptive capacity throughout the life sequence.

Though the aging process has been studied extensively no one theory has been advanced to answer all the questions raised. Since entropy seems to be one of

---

1. Simonson, E., Physiology of work capacity and fatigue, C.C. Thomas, Springfield, Ill., 1971.
2. Terris, M., Approaches to an epidemiology of health, Am. J. Public Health, Vol. 65, 1975, 1037-1045.

the premier variables in nature, which may at times parallel the direction and irreversibility of time, it appeals to many as a powerful tool in longevity analysis. Entropy is a vital concept for us; it has direct relevance in the understanding of shrinking resources, increased pollution problems and our nascent sense of social responsibility, all of which epitomize our present and will shape our future.[1] It has been applied in one form or another for 120 years. When the question of the appropriateness of entropy calculations for biological systems was submitted to an international conference at the College de France in 1938, it excited much acrimonious debate and no agreement could be reached.[2] The difficulty focused on the fact that living systems must exchange matter and energy with the environment in order to survive and hence are open systems, not in equilibrium with the environment. Prigogine and Wiame[3] published an extended form of the second law of thermodynamics which applied not only to isolated (closed) systems but also to open (and possibly living) systems. Subsequently Prigogine[4] divided entropy generation of an open system into two parts: the entropy flow due to exchanges with the surroundings (food and inspired and expired air for a living person) and the internal entropy production of irreversible (chemical, metabolic) processes. Internal entropy production is always zero (if we could live at an infinitesimally slow rate) or greater than zero (as we live normally and age irreversibly), but the external entropy exchange can have any sign, depending on what comes in and goes out of our bodies. We are open and maintain ourselves by the transfer of food and air (energy and matter) with the environment and by a continuous Dionysian chemical synthesis.[5] The metabolic rates of

1. Gatlin, L., Information theory and the living system, New York, Columbia University Press, 1972.
2. Brillouin, L., American Scientist, Vol. 37, 1949, 554.
3. Prigogine, I., J.M. Wiame, Biologie et thermodynamique des phenomenes irreversibles, Experimentia (Basel), Vol 2, 1946, 451.
4. Prigogine, I., Introduction to thermodynamics of irreversible Processes, 3rd edition, New York, Interscience, 1967.
5. Von Bertalanffy, L.V., The theory of open systems in physics and biology, Science, Vol. 111, 1950, 23-9.

living organisms of necessity must not be too slow; hence they contain a large number of irreversible processes (chemical reactions)[1] which contribute to the internal entropy production[2] and its concomitant effect, the heat evolved. Maximum entropy (disorder is at its highest level) is perhaps equivalent to senile death (not caused by accidents or any unusual intervention). It may be that death is lurking when our lifetime accumulation of entropy approaches a predetermined, fixed allocation for our species. Or when our rate of production dips to some lower critical minimum level where we are faced with a loss of vitality and are weakened sufficiently so that any one of a number of life's minor stresses (minor when we are younger) becomes a killing stress. The onset of a cold in a very old person frequently leads to pneumonia and complications which undermine the general health and vigor of the old person to the point where he or she finally succumbs.

An important advance in the study of metabolism occurred when it was demonstrated that the amount of energy liberated by the food consumed in our bodies was exactly the same as that obtained from burning the food in laboratory calorimeters.[3] This liberated energy inside of us finds its way out, to the atmosphere. Essentially all of the energy of muscle contractions in maintaining muscle tone appears as heat because little or no external work is done.[4] Energy can be stored by forming ATP; the amount of energy storage varies, but in fasting individuals it is zero or negative.[5] Therefore, in an individual who is not moving (no external work) and has not eaten recently (no energy storage), essentially all the energy output appears as heat.[6] In a resting, fasting state,

---

1. Olivera, R.J., P. Pfuderer, Test for the missynthesis of lactate dehydrogenase in aging mice by use of a monospecific antibody, Exp. Geron. Vol. 8, 1973, 193-8.
2. Hershey, D., H.H. Wang, A new age-scale for humans, Lexington Books, D.C. Heath, Lexington, Mass. 1980.
3. Kleiber, M., The fire of life, New York, Wiley, 1961.
4. Guyton, A.C., Textbook in medical physiology, 4th Ed., Philadelphia, Saunders, 1971.
5. Broda, E., The evolution of bioenergetic processes, New York, Pergamon, 1975.
6. Kleiber, M., The fire of life, New York, Wiley, 1961.

metabolic activity can be measured as the rate of heat transfer from our bodies to the surroundings. To compare metabolic rates of different persons or between species, we stipulate the experimental conditions as: complete mental and physical rest; in a room with a comfortable temperature; 12 to 14 hours after the last meal. The metabolic rate determined is ordained the basal metabolic rate (BMR); it is not the lowest value since the sleeping rate is lower. Using the prefatory word, basal, implies these specific, standard experimental conditions :

1. The subject has not been exercising for a period of 30 to 60 minutes prior to the measurement.
2. The subject is in a state of absolute mental and physical rest, but awake (the sympathetic nervous system is not overactive).
3. The subject must not have eaten anything during the last 12-to-14 hour period prior to the measurement. (Proteins need up to 14 hours to be completely metabolized.)
4. The ambient air temperature must be comfortable, 62 to 87°F (which prevents stimulation of the sympathetic nervous system).
5. The subject must have a normal body temperature of approximately 98.6°F.
6. The pulse rate and respiration must be below 80 beats per minute and 25 cycles per minute, respectively.
7. The subject should wear a loose-fitting gown to keep the same experimental conditions each time.

As discussed previously, for the human in a basal state, essentially all the energy output from the catabolism of food in the body appears as heat and the rate of internal production of entropy related to its metabolism surpasses by far that connected with other causes of irreversibility.[1] So now we know that the internal entropy production can be calculated from the heat of the chemical reactions in our bodies (divided by body temperature) and that this heat can be obtained

---
1. Prigogine, I., J.M., Wiame, Biologie et thermodyamique des phenomenes irreversibles, Experimentia, Vol. 2, 1946, 451.

from the BMR. The external entropy exchange is obtained from a knowledge of the amount and composition of the inhaled and exhaled air we breathe. The sum is our rate of entropy production. From these ideas, we find the expected lifespan for males in general is around 84 years; for females the corresponding figure is 96 years.[1] (Based on Metropolitan Life Insurance data these numbers become 103 and 109 years respectively for males and females.) If there is such a thing as a critical BMR value, we would expect this at senile death (103 or 84 years for males, depending on which set of data is used) and we find this critical BMR value to be 0.84 kilocalories per kilogram weight per hour for males (0.83 according to Calloway[2]). This translates into a critical entropy production in the vicinity of death of 0.00269 kilocalories per kilogram weight per hour per degree Kelvin temperature for men; the corresponding value for women was 0.00260. The wear and tear (rate of living) theory of aging allows that we have within us a programmed amount of life "substance" which is consumed in proportion to the duration and manner of living. When we deplete it or if the residual drops to some critical level, or the rate at which we use the elemental material diminishes to some sensitive mark, we are vulnerable to death. Hershey and Wang[3] have pooled the BMR data of the last fifty years in order to identify average, typical entropy production curves. Where the curve levels off after its steady decline with age, at age of 84 years for men, death is imminent. Prigogine and Zotin independently proposed this as the criterion of impending death: the principle of minimum entropy production. From our composite curves, the total lifetime accumulation of entropy for men and women is 2,395 and 2,551 respectively, in units of kilocalories per kilogram per degree Kelvin. This then is our potential. We can calculate your

---

1. Hershey, D., H.H. Wang, A new age-scale for humans, Lexington Books, D.C. Heath, Lexington, Mass. 1980.
2. Calloway, N.O., Heat production and senescence, Am. Geriatric Soc., Vol. 22, No. 4, 1974, 149-150.
3. Hershey, D., H.H. Wang, A new age-scale for humans, Lexington Books, D.C. Health, Lexington, 1980.

specific cumulative entropy production from birth up to a given chronological age and compare this with the average cumulative figure for a human subject. If your number is higher than average, you are living at a faster pace and are older than average since you are depleting the lifetime potential at an accelerated rate. How long you live depends on when you reach the neighborhood of 2,395 (men) or 2,551 (women).

Chapter 17

The Aging Professor

I'll tell you later about the aging professor, and how it feels to be one of them. But in those days, in the olden days when I was young I learned that students are people; so are professors. Nothing more, nothing less. Once you agree to this, then the teaching-learning process is easy. Be natural, all of you, teachers and students and many problems will be overcome. Pompous asses, brittle psyches, dishonest talk are all enemies of good teaching and effective learning. The teacher teaches, not from omniscience, and not because he is omnipotent, but because he wants to. The student learns because he has some knowledge and wishes more. The student learns because he needs to know something for his livelihood or his gratification. Teacher and student should interact, honestly, naturally, openly and in good will. Everything else is a detail. My colleague is a student. My friend is my teacher.

New teacher, old teacher: it doesn't matter. Do you stand up front and lecture or would you rather show slides? It doesn't matter. Move baby, move. Your eyes, your voice, your mind—keep them active and interesting. Laugh a little, it's not that serious. Don't you know the answer? Say so, they'll understand. "But I'll find out." "What do you think?" "Yes, that makes sense." A newly emerging professor needs to consider seriously what it takes to become a good teacher. It helps if you know your material well and have some innate interest in the subject. Beyond that there are no set rules to follow, no formulas to invoke, though there are those who will insist that this intangible, esoteric process of learning can be mechanized. A good teacher is a good person. He has basically decent instincts and respects students as persons, though we all have our imperfections, teachers and students. The good teacher avoids the extremes of attitudes: he knows that he doesn't know everything and is willing to admit that the student is not totally devoid of knowledge or sense. We can help each other. We can learn from each other.

If you are a standup lecturer, don't stand transfixed and expect the verity of your words to overcome student restlessness and the desire to be elsewhere. Man's bottom was not designed to be imprisoned in wood or plastic seats in fifty-minute intervals. Stroll around the classroom, work your way to the rear of the room, stand at the sides and challenge your students to move their eyes and necks, if for no other reason than to get a little exercise. Allow your students to exercise their vocal chords occasionally. Your lecture material has not been carried down from the mountain.

Have you seen a good movie lately? Is there some funny incident which happened to you recently? Tell about it in the classroom. Let your students in on it. They'll appreciate the respect you show for their intellect. Who knows, they may even tell you something in exchange.

A new professor becomes a good teacher when he finds his particular style of teaching, with whatever tools of the trade that suit him. He will not be embarrassed to admit that he doesn't know something, or has made a mistake. He'll be willing to find out about it and report to the class the next time. The professor has matured when he feels he has control over the dynamics of the classroom and can manipulate the various components. Large classes are handled about as well as small classes when you have enough experience. The intimacy of the small class and the informal environment are not present in the large class situation but the experienced teacher can adapt his style to the large class. He may not enjoy teaching the large class which requires a more formal, lecture-style approach but he can identify what it takes to make the large class go.

The debate surrounding large versus small classrooms pits the cost-conscious administrator against the idealist, the showman-professor against the encounter group persuader. State legislatures are for large classes, students are against them. Some professors say it doesn't make any difference whether they teach large classes or small ones, others say it cramps their style. Students are still against large classes. They sit in a hall with five-hundred kindred souls and feel lost. Their buddies are dozing or eating or standing in the rear. The teacher does not notice. They try to listen, but the echos confuse the senses. Would you like to ask a question? Don't bother, there is no time. Why hold up the progress of a teacher who is programmed to run for fifty minutes. It's unfair to the other five-hundred if you stop the lecture to get your personal question covered. Besides, how would the professor notice you—he's nearsighted. But it's so efficient to have large classes and we must be cost effective. Education must pay. It's not necessary to have a teacher—a live teacher—in the vicinity. A facimile on the television screen will do, just like the experiments with baby monkeys being mothered by bailing wire, hair and rags shaped anthropomorphically. Large classes are all right for vice presidents of universities, but they're not satisfactory to the students. The Yankee Stadium is not a classroom.

If you are a teacher, do you teach one course or two, or three or four? It makes a difference. College teaching has not yet sunk to the morale-disturbing level of grade school or high school teaching. It is not necessary to spend forty hours in a classroom to be classified as a teacher. The grade school and high school teachers are required to teach, and teach, and teach until they are sick and tired of the exercise, and become disillusioned and demoralized. They come in with high hopes, get dulled by the constant repetition and the lack of challenging scholarship and the drudgery of housekeeping chores. Though the college professor is not yet molded to this dour image, he is on the verge. The university, where scholarship and teaching are paramount, is a lovely place to be. The university professor is stimulated by his reading and research and other professional activities which sharpen his tongue in the classroom. Two or three courses each term, six to ten hours per week in the classroom, make counseling of students before and after classes not a chore but an experience. The papers the professors author, the meetings they attend, the books they write all contribute to those hours in the classroom when knowledge and experience flow unhindered. But the state legislatures are souring on the professors. "Who do they think they are? We work a full day, so should they. Keep them in the classroom where they belong. When I telephone, they better be next to the phone." So the teaching loads are creeping upward and the classrooms are getting larger. The institutions are changing and so are the experiences. Down we go.

How will I give grades in a large class? What kind of exams are made up for large classes as opposed to small ones? There is a difference. The examinations made up for large classes are formal and stylized, fill in or multiple choice, ready for easy grading by the graduate assistants who are paid to do this chore. No margin for ambiguity in these exams, don't think out of order, don't speculate beyond your nose. Give only the standard reply. No imagination needed here. Those who make up these exams cannot experiment with unusual approaches, do not introduce unorthodox ideas, dare not ask serious, deep questions. Unless the professor who produces these questions wants to grade five-hundred papers—which he doesn't. The graduate students grade the papers unhappily, impatient to do their own work but needing the money which comes in as a result of this scholarly activity. Average the grades, set them up in descending order: 90—100 is A; 80—90 is B; 70—80 is C, etc. No deviations: 89.4 is always B.

We need grades because we need order and measures of our worth. Are you an A student? Good for you, it must be better to be A than B. But A may be good at memorization and scores well on the straightforward exams of the large class. B may be unorthodox, an original thinker, turned off by the computer card mentality. It doesn't make any difference. A is better than B always. F is horrible, double jeopardy. Not only does F have to repeat the course, but he gets his cumulative average pulled down by his failure. Everything counts, everyone must get credit, even negative credit. This imperfect system can never be made ideal, but can we at least remove the double jeopardy from F? Failure means repeat of the course but why should the record include the failure. Why not have the record clean until you pass and produce something positive to show for the course? Why not?

There is, or should be, little distinction between the graduate student and the undergraduate. We have in the past attributed a quantum jump in talent, maturity and motivation to a student, the instant he received a bachelors degree and became a graduate student. There is no such gross distinction. Some undergraduates are better students than the graduate population and ought to be treated appropriately. Probably it would be better to remove the distinction altogether, eliminating such an appelation as graduate student. They, graduate and undergraduate, are students, people with likes and dislikes, talents and hangups, like all of us. Classes that have no strict prerequisites ought to be open to all students and progress measures ought to be flexible on all levels. The curricula for graduate students are usually quite arbitrary, it being supposed that these students are mature enough to wend their way through a proper program. Why not do the same for the undergraduate? We would find after a while that certain educational patterns would evolve that would be quite interesting and wholly acceptable to the professors. If graduate students do research, so can undergraduates. Let them, both groups, mingle and meet on the research and scholarship level, in the laboratory and in the classroom. The benefits for both groups of students, for the university, for the professor and the administrators would be significant. We would get educated.

Students learn from their professors, from books, from their peer groups, from their social organizations and from life. The classroom is just one avenue and this ought to be recognized. Everything cannot be told in fifty minute segments so it becomes necessary to allow the student some leeway. Ask him to read his books. Arrange assignments that require him to interact with his fellow students. Let him pick your mind in class and in your office. Talk to him—formally and informally. Give him some perspective.Experiment. Have few rigidities. Be ready to change directions when you sense that one approach is not working for this particular student or group of students. The variations are called teaching methods and are very closely related to the life style of the professor and the students. In theory, ideally, the relationship of student and professor is symbiotic.

The professor who is active in his research is more likely to be a good teacher, but not necessarily. If the researcher likes students, respects them as people, then the professor-researcher can bring to the classroom a sharpness of mind, a sense of inquiry which stimulates his approach in the classroom. He will not be content to recite the humdrum and humbug of a tired, stale curriculum, preferring to inject fresh ideas and stimulating problems from time to time. In the forefront of knowledge is where the action is, where the esoteric questions are posed and where there may not yet be any definite answers. The students in these well-taught classes grow with the professor, as he explores the unknown and admits that not all the questions of our world have been answered. The students begin to feel that they too can pose some of these marvelously exciting questions. They may even suggest some answers.

Research is a frame of mind, in that those who are actively involved are inquisitive. The researchers also publish their results, for many reasons. There is of course the ego factor, in seeing your name in print. Your colleagues around the country admire you, know your name and invite you to be chairman of symposia. Job offers also result from publishing, and so do simple invitations to speak at other schools. Within your own university augmented salary and promotions may result from significant publications. So the researcher publishes, actively, until he has secured his position in his field and his university. Thereafter he publishes only what he truly likes, casting off the marginal material that he would have published in his younger days.

Teaching a college class is similar to performing on stage in the show business world. Your audience is up front; you enter the arena with a script and begin the show. Some teachers are dull performers, with no confidence to digress from the script. These insecure teachers copy the material from their notes onto the blackbord. The students in turn "take notes", which means that they recopy the information, this time from the blackboard into their notebooks. Such is the flow of knowledge in a dull class. On the other hand, there is the professor who has taught his subject so frequently that he has no need in class to refer to a textbook or his notes. This teacher leaves his reference material in his office and strides confidently, seemingly naked, into the classroom. It is a wonder to behold, and quite often the professor can put on a sterling show. He roams all over the classroom, gesticulates, varies his inflections and analyzes his students as a quarterback would examine the opposition's defensive formations in football. But we may also pity this professor. If he has taught the same course so frequently, in the same manner, with the same material, for so long that he needs no notes, then this teacher must be stagnating in his field. Most professors come into the class with some notes or a textook and proceed with a combination of oral exposition and blackboard writing to cause knowledge to flow from a region of high concentration to one of low concentration. This is scientifically possible, according to the second law of thermodynamics, but the professors don't always succeed.

A new teacher has to decide on the textbooks to be used for his courses, which means he has read the various books before the beginning of the term so he can have some perspective with respect to the philosophy and train of thought of the authors. (In the sciences it's also desirable to solve some of the homework problems beforehand in order to know what problems are available and how difficult they would be for the students.) A novice professor can't easily estimate how much material will be required in order to fill a one-hour class, nor is he sure what teaching style is suited to his personality. Giving quizzes rather than taking them is also a new experience for him and consequently becomes another unknown factor. All of these worries are superimposed upon a general feeling of insecurity.

"Do I really know more than they do?"

As unprepared as he imagines that he is, the new teacher does manage to get ready for the first class, sweating a little under the armpits in the process. Finally in he goes to that first class containing all those unfamiliar and critical faces. But for the new professor, the most difficult and soul-searching problems arise at the end of the course, when he must quantitatively evaluate the students and give out grades. The initial steps are easy for the teacher, as he sums the examination scores of each student, calculating the individual averages and arranging these averages in descending order. Now begins the perplexing job. Who deserves an A grade? How many students should get A's? Is it clear where the separation is between A and B? If he is fortunate, the teacher will find an abrupt separation between the A group and the rest of the students. Most likely there will not be a clear-cut demarcation and so he must decide, on the basis of insufficient evidence, which students are to get the A grades. And then he must deal with the remaining names on the list. He culls the B students, then the C students and soon the most unpleasant task is before him. Is anyone to fail? Is there an obvious distinction in average grade between the bottom group and the others? (Sometimes there is but most often there is not.) Should the bottom group get F grades? Now he must play God.

Perhaps for the first time in his life this new teacher has conscious, significant control over the destiny of people who have no personal involvement with him. If the incipient F student failed to do the work required, and in other ways conveyed a lack of accomplishment and interest, then the decision to "award" this student an F will not be so difficult. But if this marginal student did make a serious effort to learn and was apparently interested in the course and the manner by which you taught it, then the giving of an F grade will be a painful act. The decision tears at the thin veneer of self-confidence which a new professor constructs.

"Is it I or the student who failed?" he thinks uncomfortably.

"Is it my teaching technique that was a failure?"

"Were my exams fair?"

"Am I prejudiced in some way?"

Ultimately the new professor makes the required decisions and goes on to the next class, but the uncertainty nags at him.

To be a virgin assistant professor is to be hung upon two dilemmas which set up excruciating tensions. On the one hand, you are a hot-shot, a new boy in town, a source of the latest information, full of energy, and embodying all those powerful traits of the young. You express a natural empathy for the student, enjoying a common ethos. On the other hand, you gaze upon your elders and marvel at the years of experience, the papers published, the books written, the cool elan generated by their sense of belonging and controlling.

I wondered how shall I ever know as much as they, while at the same time, I was ready to be better than they ever were. It is the way of life for the younger, more vigorous, to strive for success, to overcome, to be equal to their elders and perhaps surpass their accomplishments. But what is an old professor? How is the transition made, from young to old? What is an old teacher? An old researcher? An old hand at committee work? Are you a smarter professor in your old age? Do you really know more? Can you teach better?

I am not yet old, but I have begun to understand the implication of these questions. When young, I worked long hours alone, paying very close attention to detail—every detail—trying to be perfect. My brain was tested constantly, its circuits stimulated and buzzing, generating those beautiful, original thoughts. Read, study, derive those equations, learn new things, incorporate everything into a grand design. The result was innovative, exciting teaching and research. And now in my second decade as a professor I realize that I too am not equal to my youth. There are compensating ways, though, for the maturing professor learns that the path to success isn't necessarily a direct, naked attack on ignorance, rather a controlled production of a portfolio which reflects his accomplishments and philosophy.

The middle-aged professor such as I, with the burst of youthful energy dissipated, now finds fewer intellectual peaks and valleys. There is less time for total immersion in my work, for among other reasons, vitality is diminished, and diverting responsibilities of family and community take their toll. So I skim more, allowing my eyes to race over the pages of journals and books, searching for key words and phrases which touch an academic nerve. My research interests are narrowing.

The aging professor spends less time on research, more time in the evenings reading for enjoyment, less time preparing class lectures, more time with his family, less time publishing papers and books, more time sleeping, less time in the classroom, more time on vacation, less time discussing his speciality with his colleagues, more time on committees, less time on brain-stressing problem-solving, more time on community projects. The aging professor seems to hang onto the old-fashioned ideas of his field, appears to be obsolescent and unable or unwilling to adduce the new trends, the latest techniques, the most recent theories or points of view. He is conservative, more conservative than in his youth, more fearful of change, more determined to maintain the status quo, as things were in the halcyon days of the ivory tower. The old professor feels he is becoming a Neanderthal, becoming one of those dinosaurs. I too have begun to have these feelings. I sense that my background is becoming inadequate, but I counter this by asking: inadequate for what? My students possess the skills I no longer command. Oh, I can learn these things, if I wish, but there is not time, I tell myself. We've heard this refrain before, haven't we? I suppose each of us feels his case is the exception.

But what does the old professor feel in his sixth decade of life? Was he a mediocre professor? Was his teaching poor? Was the material presented in his courses too elementary? Was his research non-existent? What does he think about, now within a few years of retirement? Was it all worthwhile? Did he need to become an academic type and expose his deficiencies so publicly? Gone is the expectation or hope of contributing significantly to the development of his field, or of becoming famous. And it is no longer possible to begin anew, to develop another professional interest. It is too late for now he has too many grey whiskers. His early habits are now cast in stone, the delicate machinery is fused and sluggish. How do you change an old organism? They say you can't teach an old dog new tricks; a given input yields a predictable output. He ought to know this, so cut out the bullshit and ask him to resign from the human race.

How unfair to think this. What good is the old professor? Can he make a contribution? To the university? To himself? Let's salvage him. With his years of experience, he has some acquired traits and knowledge which we can mashall and focus. Can we find a way which will allow this old professor to regain some self-esteem, to be "pumped up" in his old age so that he will not fall into the human garbage heap? We owe it to him, as you will some day owe it to me. We shall say to him: What are you good at? What do you want to do? How do you wish to be remembered? What is important to you? And then we shall ask him to fulfill his mission, to aspire once again. To reactivate the dormant blood vessels and nerve endings of his human fiber, to become young again in spirit, to plan, to think, to strive to be a person of some value. There are those who will scoff, who will say it is not worth the effort. Force him to retire to make room for the younger person. They will say that rejuvenation is impossible. I will respond by saying it is worth the time and effort if we can salvage the old professor who is a human being.

Chapter 18

Cities, Corporations, Civilizations: Size; Structure; Stability; Senescence

Calculations of entropy changes in open systems were reported in 1896, entropy production in 1911.[1] Clausius coined the word, entropy, from the Greek language to mean transformation and defined it as the increment of energy added to a body as heat divided by its temperature, during a reversible process. Brillouin showed a connection between entropy and information.[2] Dowds[3] developed his own method of applying entropy concepts to the examination of the data from oil fields, as did others in land use planning and in prediction of travel between different communities[4] and in Nigeria to analyze water runoff.[5] It was the work of Shannon[6] that more firmly connected information and entropy. If information is being sent, it must be possessed by the sender and we can speak of the probability of a message being sent. Suppose entropy measures not the information of the sender but the ignorance of the receiver—removed by the

---

1. Wisonewski, B., B. Staniozewskis, R. Syzmanik, Thermodynamics of nonequilibrium proceses, Boston, Riedel, 1979, 21.
2. Tribus, M., Thirty years of information theory, in The maximum entropy formalism, Levine, R.D., M. Tribus, editors, The MIT Press, Cambridge, Mass., 1978.
3. Dowds, J.P., Application of information theory in establishing oil field trends, in Computers in the mineral industries, Parks, G.A., Editor, Stanford U. Press, 1964.
4. Wilson, A.G., The use of entropy maximizing models in the theory of trip distribution, mode split and route split, J. Transport Economics and Policy, Jan., 1969.
5. Sonuga, J.O., Entropy principle applied to rainfall runoff process, J. Hydrology, Vol. 30, 1976, 81-94.
6. Shannon, C., W. Weaver, The mathematical theory of communications, U. Illinois Press, Urbana, 1949.

receipt of the message. The probabilities assigned individual messages are a means of describing a state of knowledge. Historians such as Toynbee, Spengler and Spencer who believed in historical determinism, reified civilizations, associating them with the living tendencies of birth, maturation, senility and death. The question is whether entropy and information theory can be applied to corporations, countries and civilizations.

Shannon's formula connects informational entropy to the probability that the system is in a certain structural configuration.[1,2] A number from one to one hundred can always be identified in seven guesses (which can be answered by yes or no). To do this one needs to make guesses in such a way as to eliminate one-half of the remaining range. By applying Shannon's formula we can calculate the informational entropy for this process; we get the number of guesses required to find the unknown number, or the amount of entropy information associated with the process. The relationship between entropy and information provides further clarification of the fundamental principle of the living process: increases in entropy can be viewed as a destruction of information. A living, open organism must be able to maintain its organized state against the forces of disorganization; it must continue homeostasis and a purposeful behavior.

Disturbed slightly, we will return to the same steady state conditions as soon as the tampering ceases. Body temperature is an example of such behavior; with the invasion of foreign organisms, the antibody-antigen reaction results in a raising of the temperature set point and we develop a fever. When the external influences diminish, we return to our normal temperature. If however small departures from the steady state are magnified so that the system moves even further away, the steady state is unstable. There may be several steady states or plateaus, as suggested by Prigogine: stability

---

1. Rapoport, A., Lewis, F. Richardson's mathematical theory of war, General Systems, Vol. XXIII, 1978, 67-103.
2. Rapoport, A., Mathematical aspects of general analysis, General Systems, XXIII, 1978, 139-147.

through fluctuations. The more the system is organized (in our youth), the more it is equipped to resist killing stresses, a situation reversed in old age when there is more disorganization and less ability to resist disturbances which overcome our stability criteria. In the theory of social systems many analogies suggest themselves; the institution can be easily imagined to be an organism.[1] It's organizational structure can be thought to correspond to our anatomy, it's modus operandi to physiology, its history to our development and evolution. Mathematical models of power relations among states have been drawn to help clarify the distinction between stable and unstable states. If states in concert and vying with each other for power constitute a system, then the system also has certain properties of stability. Economic systems are also included here; to the extent that certain aspects of an economic system (fluctuations in production levels, prices, or investment capital) can be cast in a mathematical model, questions about equilibrium, stability and instability can be answered by mathematical deduction rather than by intuitive guesses. The models are based on the assumption that there can be transitions of a system from state to state, governed somewhat by probabilities. In a large population, probabilities become frequency of occurence.

In the matter of nation systems, size may govern stability.[2] A nation becomes too big when it can no longer provide its citizens with the services they expect—defense, roads, health, courts, etc.—without amassing such complicated institutions and bureacracies that they actually end up preventing the very goals they are attempting to achieve, a phenomenon common in the world today. The notion that size governs is one that has long been familiar; Haldane showed many years ago that if a mouse were to be as large as an elephant, it would have to become an elephant, that is, it would have to develop those features such as heavy, stubby legs to allow it to

---

1. Rapoport, A., Mathematical aspects of general analysis, General Systems, XXIII, 1978, 139-147.
2. Kohr, L., The breakdown of nations, Dutton, New York, 1978.

support its weight. City planners realize that accumulations of people much above 100,000 create entirely new problems: it is virtually impossible for a city exceeding this size to run in the black since the municipal services it must supply cost more than any feasible amount of taxation can raise. Social problems expand at a geometric ratio with the growth of a city while the ability to cope with them expands only arithmetically. Nuclear explosions result when a certain critical mass is reached. Cancer represents a group of cells outgrowing their normal bounds. Isn't it true that human beings, charming in small aggregations, become mobs when overconcentrated. The problem then may be how to stop growing: division when size becomes overbearing. Arnold Toynbee, linking the downfall of civilizations not to the fight amongst nations but to the rise of universal (large) states, suggests that we return to the Greek ideal of a self-regulatory balance of small units.[1] Kathleen Freeman[2] in a study of Greek City-States shows that nearly all Western culture is the product of the disunited small states of ancient Greece and that these same states produced almost nothing after they became united under Rome. Justice Brandeis[3] devoted a lifetime to exposing bigness by demonstrating that beyond relatively narrow limits, additional growth of plant or organizational size no longer adds to, but detracts from the efficiency and productivity of firms. Henry Simmons[4] asserts the obstacles to world peace do not lie in the alleged anachronisms of little states but in the great powers and suggests their dismantlement. Kohr claims the principal immediate cause behind both the regularly recurring outbursts of mass criminality and the accompanying moral numbness does not seem to lie in a perverted leadership or corrupt philosophy but is linked with frequency and numbers, which are intensifiers and with the possession of the critical quantity of power—which has a

---

1. Toynbee, A.J., A study of history, Oxford U. Press, New York, 1972.
2. Freeman, K., Greek City-States, New York, W.W. Norton, 1950.
3. Brandeis, L.D., The curse of bigness, New York, Viking, 1935.
4. Simmons, H.C., Economic policy for a free society, Chicago, U. of Chicago Press, 1948.

detonating effect. In a small society, the critical quantity of power can only rarely accumulate since the cohesive force of the group is easily immobilized by self-balancing centrifugal trends of individuals. In evaluating the critical size of a society, it is not sufficient to think only in terms of the size of its population. Density and the velocity of information flow (related to the extent of its administrative integration and technological progress) must likewise be taken into account. A large population thinly spread may act as a small society. Similarly, a volatile and faster moving society may transgress the bounds into an unstable state: an agitated crowd in a theater may tax the heretofore adequate number of exits. Larger—excessively large—communities require saturation police forces to match at all times the latent power of the community. The numbers are simple to handle in small social units. The answer to the problem may reside not in increased police power but in a reduction of social size—the dismemberment of those units of society that have become too big. Aggression, in countries as well as communities, arises spontaneously, irrespective of nationality or disposition, the moment the power becomes so great that in the estimation of its leaders the system has outgrown the power of its prospective adversaries. We should strive for the opposite of the unification or one-world principle. The recusants say it is ridiculous to maintain that a small-state world would eliminate wars. What about the dark Middle Ages during which both small states and uninterrupted wars prevailed? Kohr in rebuttal points out that the wars were of considerably smaller magnitude and were fought over less consequential matters than we face today; small wars fought by small states were the usual, expected perturbations. Even today. Civilization was not threatened. Great powers produced great, world wars. In miniature, problems lose both their terror and significance which is all that society can ever hope for. The United States is internally not an uneasy assembly of great powers but of small states. As a result we benefit from the flexibility that characterizes small-cell organisms, rendering them capable of adaptation to quotidian changes in human and social conditions.

Below a certain size, everything fuses, joins or accumulates; beyond the optimal size, everything collapses or explodes (stars, atoms, etc.). The stars in the sky may seem huge, but what are they in relation to space itself? They sometimes grow to the point where instead of generating energy, they begin to absorb it (as great powers do in the political universe). The effort to maintain their existence forces these stars to consume more than they receive[1], living off their capital until the supply of hydrogen becomes exhausted. The stars collapse and in the process of collapsing generate rotary forces comparable with gravity, causing fantastic explosions as they disintegrate: the supernova. There is instability of the microcosm also, but it seems to be of minor consequence compared to the gigantic state. Being too-small leads to a self-regulating device through aggregations or fusions until a proper and stable size is achieved and the functions determined or teleological form is fulfilled.[2] Human aggregations must have magnitudes drawn from our inherent stature, and be measured in miles and years, not parsecs and eternities. For us, disease and aging produce an upset in our rhythm of life. What was previously flexible and swift now is slow and rigid. Big-power systems also move and live, though like an old person, at a reduced speed, with the accumulation of turgid or inert bulk. Every time a movement occurs in an overaged social system, a powerful authority is required to rearrange its obdurate, unified cells in a new balance. Hence the fanatical attempts of our statesman to create super-governments in the form of the League of Nations and the United Nations. No longer able to do what small, more flexible states could, the superpower world, unable to govern itself, looks for an external controlling agent. A good balance of systems in the world, be it of stars, states or people must be flexible and self-

---

1. Hoyle, F., The nature of the universe, Oxford, Basil Blackwell, 1950.
2. Thompson, D'Arcy, W., On growth and form, London, Cambridge University Press, 1942.

regulatory, derived from the independent existence of a great number of small-component parts held together not in tight unity but elastic harmony. If opportunism, necessary to living systems, deteriorates as a result of overgrown cells, then it follows that we may restore proper function through cell division and the reintroduction of a small-cell arrangement. Division represents a cure principle and progress while unification seems to portend disease and primitivism. Language conveys more information through a division of sounds. Parties may be saved from boredom not by having all guests assembled in a single circle dominated by a magnetic personality, but by dissolving the pattern of unity into a number of small groups. By branching off into a number of different forms, orders, classes and subclasses, an originally unified group diversifies itself. The first step towards a higher form of life was accomplished when living substances differentiated into green plants, bacteria, fungi and animals.[1] If large bodies are inherently unstable in the physical universe, they are in all likelihood unstable also in the social universe. What is applicable in the universe as a whole and in special fields such as biology, engineering and art should also be appropriate in politics.[2] The law of crowded living is in other words, organization; the greater the aggregation, the more dwarfish we become. But what is the ideal size of a state? Up to what point can a political community grow without endangering the existence of the state and the individual? Or how small can it become before we achieve a similar denouement? When does a community become stable? And for how long? The early Greek, Italian or German city-states contained ten or twenty thousand people. With a population of less than a hundred-thousand, Salzburg produced churches, a university, several other schools of higher learning and half a dozen theaters. Plato thought a population of 5,040 was best; Thomas More's towns in Utopia held 6,000 families. Robert Owens parallelograms comprised 500 to 2,000

---

1. Huxley, J., Biological improvement, The Listener, Nov. 1, 1951, 739.
2. Kohr, L., op. cited, 97.

members and Horace Greeley's associations were to number from some hundreds to thousands of persons. William Morris envisaged a return to a society from which all big cities had disappeared and London dissolved into a number of villages separated by woods.[1] Small states with their concise dimensions and relatively insignificant problems of communal living gives their citizens time and leisure, without which no great art can develop; large powers with their enormous social demands consume practically all the available energy of their servants and citizens, in the mere task of keeping their immobile, clumsy societies functioning. Forever afraid of cracking beneath their own oppressive weight, gigantic states can never release their populations from servitude to their collective enterprise. They are deflected from the grace of individual living to the puritan virtue of cooperation. which is the law of some highly efficient animal societies. Arnold Toynbee in his A Study of History[2] suggested a consanguity between cultural productivity and relief from exacting social tasks in nations, states and churches. What is great in great nations is not to be found during their periods of power (which kept them busy with occupying the limelight on the stage of history) but during the time when they were relatively insignificant and little. In the large state we are forced to live in tightly specialized compartments where life's experiences are carefully circumscribed, whose borders we almost never cross. According to Kohr, the great empires of antiquity, including the Roman Empire have not created a fraction of the culture which the ever-feuding Greek city-states produced. The great empires' chief accomplishments were technical and social, not cultural.[3] They had administrators, strategists and road builders, their cultural accomplishments were derived from the members of small disunited and quarrelsome tribes whom they bought on the slave markets. England produced the glittering list of

---

1. Kohr, L., op. cited, 107-8.
2. Toynbee, A.J., A study of history, New York, Oxford U. Press, 1947, 224.
3. Kohr, L., op. cited, 125.

Shakespeare, Marlowe and Ben Johnson in literature when small; as England grew mightier, the nation's talents were diverted into the fields of war, administration, colonization economics. Italy and Germany were small-state systems up to about 1870 (split into little principalities, duchies, republics and kingdoms). They gave the world Dante, Michaelangelo, Raphael, Goethe, Kant, Durer, Beethoven and Bach to name a few. When the small interstate strife ceased among Italian and German principalities and republics, they began to cultivate imperial ambitions and forgot about their great intellects and artists. Culture is the product not of peoples but individuals and apparently creative persons have difficulty flourishing in the decorous atmosphere of large powers; where order and consolidation and uniformity of purpose are carried to their logical conclusion, cultural fertility withers. Toynbee in his studies of the rise and decline of civilizations[1] has portrayed a relationship between political unification and intellectual decay. He theorized a last stage of a civilization, characterized by forcible political unification into a universal state. He cites as examples: the integration of the Hellenic society into the Roman Empire; the Hindu civilization which had its universal state in the Mughal Empire and its successor, the British Raj; the Far-Eastern civilization in the Mongol Empire. Toynbee suggested the establishment of a world order of smaller states. Even in economics, unification requires the application of a system such as capitalism or socialism on too vast a scale for it to be successful. The cracks which develop in the systems are not necessarily the result of social shortcoming, but of infection whose etiology is derived from monopolies and unsurveyable, huge market areas. In order to meet our essential needs, we produce factories and their accuterments which satisfy no direct human want but have become necessary in order to enable us to meet our increasing needs. Is it the particular economic system at fault or sheer economic size? Do we outgrow our human bounds and begin to

---

1. Toynbee, A.J., op. cited, 244.

suffer from problems of unmanageable proportions? When this happens to a community, do its problems magnify, achieving a new order of demi-god dimensions, arising not from the process of living but from the business of growing. The larger more powerful societies find more of their products devoured by the task of coping with the murrain of its power. The more it gains in density, the more energy is required to survive. So we build the bombs and tanks and the military budget rises disproportionately. And so do the welfare costs, traffic lights, auto accidents, parking lots, etc. Business cycles, attributed mostly to capitalistic countries are nevertheless phenomena also of socialistic systems; the problem is not the ideology. Once beyond a certain size, it becomes increasingly difficult to deal with economic pertubations, the cycle of boom and bust. The overshoot and undershoot of the cycles seem to become more closely linked to each preceding cycle and we tend towards instability—seemingly unable to dampen the fluctuations. Are we then headed for what Prigogine, in an essentially optimistic vein, has called stability through fluctuations or are we marching towards disaster? The performance of a corporation after it has reached a certain size begins to decline in relation to the amount of resources put into it, in spite of the illusionary fact that the total output may continue to increase. Wise businessmen will not extend production to maximum capacity but to optimum capacity. Instead we should build new and independent plants and begin the battle against diminishing productivity again, but now with a small-cell model; a sound capitalist economy should be founded on individual diversity: "care is taken that the trees do not scrape the skies".[1] Corporations grouped as medium sized or small had lower average costs of production or higher rates of return on invested capital than their large-sized counterparts.[2]

---

1. Brandeis, L.D., op. cited, 117.
2. Anonymous, Temporary National Economic Committee, Relative efficiency of large, medium-size and small businesses, Monograph No. 13, Washington Govt. Printing Office, 1941, 10.

In a small-cell organization, superiority of federal power over its strongest unit is easily accomplished because even the strongest unit is weak. On the other hand large cells are difficult to dominate: the costs of the necessary police force could be prohibitive and members of these cells may be reluctant to contribute funds for an umbrella organization capable of overshadowing their own position. To enforce its laws in the U.S., Washington needs only to be stronger than the most powerful or influential. California, Texas and New York seem great compared to Rhode Island but are individually less significant than the whole of the United States. The success of Switzerland as a small-cell country is not that it is a federation of three nationalities, but that it is an assembly of twenty-two states. The German federal experiment disintegrated with the expulsion of Austria in 1866, for then we saw a unification of the smaller German states with the victorious colossus, Prussia. Powerful Prussia then dominated the government; indeed the federation centralized and became the instrument of Prussian will. The Medes and Persians built history's first great exemplary model of a centralized empire by splitting their conquests into numerous small satrapies whose domination was relatively simple.[1] Alexander's empire, which failed to apply this concept, needed him to keep it together and promptly collapsed after his death. The Romans centralized their dominion, dividing their vast and long-lasting holdings into small controllable provinces in which no countervailing power could develop to hinder the work of the Roman proconsuls. Divide and rule. Napoleon dissolved France's large duchies such as Burgundy into more than ninety small departments. The new units had no history, no disruptive hatreds, no competing ambitions. And no power to obstruct the rule of the central government intent upon ruling a maximum area with a minimum of means. Successful social organisms, be they empires, states, countries, cities or corporations seem to have in all their diversity of language, customs, traditions and governing systems one

---
1. Kohr, L., op. cited, 186.

common feature: the small-cell pattern. Wherever, because of age or poor design, the rejuvenation process of such division gives way to the calcifying process of cell unification, the cells (now growing beyond reasonable limits, protected by carapaced structures) develop arrogant great-power complexes which are difficult to neutralize without the drastic surgery of conquest and the restoration of the small-cell pattern.[1]

This behavior of nations and other human organizations illustrates the recondite dynamics of the nonequilibrium open system, a real world application of the theory. States, living cells, economic processes, ecological systems, transportation networks: we can create the bridges between the physical and social sciences. Prigogine is attempting to draw consistent mathematical analogies between chemical systems, entropy and social processes; Georgescu-Roegen is doing the same for economics. Prigogine studies self-organization under conditions of fluctuations and change, an evolutionary process in systems pushed far from equilibrium. Whether the fluctuations impinge on a household or a nation, the belief is that they can be explained. He examines oscillating phenomena and seeks a basis for predicting order from the perspective of entropy production (regarded by some as the reification of the arrow of time since it describes in general the direction spontaneous processes must go). Use of the term, entropy, is derived from the Greek, meaning evolution.[2] Systems near equilibrium can be buffeted by small perturbations in energy and mass pressures but no new organizations, no new structures are formed. Imposing stronger gradients from the outside world could force the appearance of new, dissipative, nonequilibrium states. Examples cited by Prigogine are a town and the living cell. Georgescu-Roegen wants economics, which ignores entropy, to begin to mark the existence and applicability of nonequilibrium dynamics and irreversibility. Economists, he says, have a

---

1. Kohr, L., op. cited, 187.
2. Lepkowski, W., The social thermodynamics of Ilya Prigogine, Chem. and Eng. News, April 16, 1979, 31.

a blind faith in reversibility (we can restore original conditions by invoking the same laws, backwards and forwards and ignoring time). Matter is subjected to entropy degradation, from higher order to lesser, and hence becomes less useful. What Georgescu-Roegen is stressing is an evolutionary philosophy. If driven hard enough we see new structures developing, nurtured by energy and matter fluxes.[1] Entropy, applied to the economic process, adds important new perceptions to the interactions of humans, technology, the market system and limited resources. Ideas spawned by Georgescu-Roegen. He proposes we think in terms of irreversibilities, limits on resource availability and a more parsimonious society. Most current economic policy tinkers with prices, taxes or the market in some way. Until now, we have stressed economic balances of energy and matter—what comes in must equal what goes out—rather than an understanding that something is lost in every transaction (in entropy terms), in transforming raw materials or energy. The real world dictates the transformation in one direction only: low entropy to high entropy. The consumer takes in high-grade, ordered energy and matter and exhausts low-grade, disordered wastes. The wastes must not injure or render inoperative the feedback and control mechanisms which affect the stability of the open, temporary state. Consumers may be individuals, cities, governments, corporations, civilizations.[2] The entropy-economics link can be applied to feasibility studies in the recovery of old oil wells, accounting and cash flow, agriculture, new product development, decision-making and information flow. Money constitutes the economic equivalent of low entropy.

Biological systems maintain a state of high coherence, which is perhaps the most striking feature of living things. They may evolve to new, temporarily

---

1. Procaccio, J., The Nobel prize in chemistry, Science, vol. 198, Nov. 18, 1977, 716-7.
2. Lepkowski, W., Researchers, policy makers relate entropy concepts to economics, Chem. and Eng. News, Nov. 14, 1977, 18-9.

organized states called dissipative structures[1,2], to signify that they are created and maintained by the dissipative, entropy-producing processes within the system: regulatory processes at the cellular level[3-6]; excitable biological systems[7-8]; cell communication and development[9]; evolution[10] and model building.[11] Viewed as a succession of instabilities within a fundamentally irreversible, self-organizing domain, the changes are achieved spontaneously, according to their own time or age scale. Some believe evolution proceeds this way; each step is followed by another which has a greater chance to occur (and hence takes less time to appear). Autocatalysis. In order to describe the behavior of a self-organizing system we need some index of the intensity of energy dissipation which will provide us with a clue as to its organizing proclivity.

Describing self-organizing processes requires us to define and quantify the notion of order; we need a model to account for the transition from one slot in the hierarchy to the next. The degree of organization of a biological system is established teleologically (with respect to its purpose): seeing from an eye, hearing from an ear, etc. The better its purpose is realized, the more organized is the system. We need criteria to characterize biological order; we need to explain the existence of selection pressures which account for the advantages gained when our purpose is realized

---

1. Glansdorf, P., I. Prigogine, Thermodynamics of structure, stability and fluctuations, Wiley-Interscience, New York, 1971.
2. Prigogine, I., G. Nicolis, Quart. Rev. Biophys., vol. 4, 1971, 107.
3. Goldbeter, A., R. Lefever, Biophys. J., vol. 12, 1972, 1302.
4. Goldbeter, A., Proc. Nat. Acad. Sci. (USA), vol. 70, 1973, 3255.
5. Babloyantz, A., G. Nicolis, J. Theoret. Biol., vol. 39, 1972, 185.
6. Babloyantz, A., M. Sanglier, F.E.B.S. Letters, vol. 23, 1972, 364.
7. Lefever, R., J.P. Changeux, C.R. Acad. Sci. (Paris), vol. 275D, 1972, 591.
8. Blumenthal, R., J.P. Changeus, R. Lefever, J. Membr. Biol., vol. 2, 1970, 351.
9. Martinez, H., J. Theoret. Biol., vol. 36, 1972, 479.
10. Prigogine, I., G. Nicolis, A. Babloyantz, Physics Today, Nov-Dec, 1972.
11. Nicolis, G., I. Prigogine, Proc. Nat. Acad. Sci. (USA), vol. 68, 1972, 2102.

with greater efficiency.[1,2] The index for evolution may be entropy production[3] and the level of interactions with the outside world. There are probabilities we can assign to the occurence of no event and, on the other hand, to one event. In other words we can use the number one or zero, to represent the fact that the event has, or has not, happened. This number, one or zero conveys exactly one bit of information (bit: a contraction of the words binary and digit). A binary number provides an amount of information which is equal to the entropy of the process generating the event. The information transmitted links to the change in the state of organization of the system. For example, during the first stage of oil exploration, an oil company will determine that one of its new wells will or will not produce oil.[4] In the second stage, the directors of the company will or will not vote a dividend. We can define probabilities in terms of (1) success in finding oil and a dividend is paid; (2) success and no dividend is paid; (3) no success in finding oil and a dividend is paid and (4) no success and no dividend is paid. We can measure the information (in entropy units) available in terms of these probabilities and ask how much information has been gained through the knowledge that the well was successful, calculated from Shannon's formula.[5]

Decentralization is a process by which decision-making authority is delegated down the organizational hierarchy. The effectiveness of such decentralization is adduced from the levels at which decision-making authority are placed and the relative importance of the decisions. We can locate the center of decision-making authority within an organization; but we are also concerned with the dispersion of the decision-makers, this

---

1. Eigen, M., Naturwiss, vol. 58, 1971, 465.
2. Kuhn, H., in Synergetics, Haken, H., B.G. Teubner, editors, Stuttgart, 1973.
3. Prigogine, I., Etude thermodynamique des phenomenes irreversibles, Paris, Dunod and Liege, Desoer, 1947.
4. Murphy, R.E., Adaptive processes in economic systems, Academic Press, New York, 1965, 74.
5. Shannon, C., W. Weaver, The mathematical theory of communication, Illinois U. Press, Urbana, Ill., 1962.

being part of the index of decentralization.[1-3] Entropy is a useful measure of dispersion and decentralization, where entropy of an organization is defined as the probability of a decision being made multiplied by the logarithm of that probability.[4] Summing these numbers over all levels of the organization is what is called Shannon's entropy formula, the uncertainty index in decision-making. If all decisions were made at one level of an organization there would be no uncertainty as to where decisions originate: an example of complete concentration of decision-making authority. Alternatively, the greatest uncertainty would occur when it was equally likely that a decision could be made at any level of the organization (a maximum dispersion of decision-making). Entropy calculated from Shannon's formula is increased when the uncertainty of a situation also increases (more dispersion of decision-making authority), attaining a maximum when all probabilities are equal. Here the probability is one in m, where m is the number of levels in the organization.[5] Entropy and dispersion may increase as the number of levels, m, of the organization is raised. The difficulty with using Shannon's formula of course resides in the stygian problem of finding the probability that a decision is rendered at a given level. If everyone is independent, we can relate probabilities to frequencies—how often decisions are made at each level and then use entropy as a measure of dispersion in the analysis of business and economic data. Hildenbrand and Paschen[6] were early believers in entropy in the analysis of economic data,

---

1. Murphy, D.C., J.T. Hasenjaeger, Entropy as a measure of decentralization, Proc. of Fifth Ann. Meet. of Amer. Inst. Decision Sciences, Boston, Nov. 14-16, 1973.
2. Baker, H., A. France, Centralization and decentralization in industrial relations, Princeton, N.J., Industrial Relations Sect. Meet. Princeton U., 1954.
3. Horwitz, A., I. Horwitz, Entropy, markov processes and competition, J. Industrial Economcis, XVI, July, 1968.
4. Thiel, H., Economics and information theory, Amsterdam, North Holland, 1967.
5. Murphy, D.C., J.T. Hasenjaeger, op. cited, 67.
6. Hildenbrand, W., H. Paschen, Ein axiomatisch begrundeites konzentrationmass, Statistical Information, Statistical Office of the European Communities, No. 3, 1964, 153-61.

using it as a measure of industrial concentration, though Thiel[1] applied it more extensively to industry sales, foreign trade and corporation balance sheets. Thus should the calculations yield an entropy value for imports of leading commodities of 2.76 for 1950 and 2.86 for 1960, we may conclude that disorder in the distribution of imports increased during this decade or that there was greater equality (likelihood) of importing food, petroleum, paper, etc. In the investment field we could assign a probability that various securities might yield given returns over a period of time and compute by Shannon's formula the entropy distribution of stock prices. Or how is world trade distributed among countries. How are assets distributed on a balance sheet? The results of these calculations have been interpreted syncretically as signifying a freedom of choice, uncertainty, disorder, information content and information gains or losses. A popular use of entropy is in the analysis of market structure[2,3,4] where in a monopoly situation where the buyer has no choice as to the firm to be patronized, the lack of choice is reflected in the entropy measure (a value of zero for a perfect monopoly). In a two-firm duopoly situation—equal sized companies—the random buyer is equally likely to patronize either firm and has only one decision: to buy from one or the other. Shannon's formula would in this case yield a number equal to 1.0. With four firms of equal size, a quadopoly, the random buyer has two dichotomous decisions: first, whether to buy from group 1 (two firms) or group 2 (two firms) and second, which firm within a group to deal with. The entropy number we calculate here is 2.0. Extending our thinking to 8 equal-sized companies, an octopoly, requires three dichotomous decisions. Where the businesses are of unequal size, the more unequal they are, the smaller the entropy value. In these calculations, entropy equates with the average number of dichotomous

---

1. Thiel, H., op. cited.
2. Finkelstein, M.O., R.M. Freidberg, The application of an entropy theory of concentration to the Clayton Act, The Yale Law Review, Vol. 76, 1976, 677-717.
3. Horwitz, A., R.I. Horwitz, op. cited, 196-211.
4. Theil, H., op. cited.

decisions the buyer must make, where the goal is to minimize the number of decisions. It becomes the degree of uncertainty as to which firm is to be chosen by the random customer. As such, entropy reflects the degree of competition. Entropy has been used in accounting, to quantify the putative loss of information when items in a financial statement are combined.[1,2,3] The entropy difference before and after combining a pair of entries tells us something about the information loss in aggregation. Information here means the elimination of uncertainty as to which of several messages has been transmitted. Or the freedom of choice we have in selecting a particular message from a set of all possible messages. Entropy is a measure of information in the sense that it focuses on the uncertainty surrounding a transmitted message. The problem of aggregation in accounting and in financial analysis is primarily that of providing the user with sufficient insight into the financial condition of the firm or the market. Rearranging and combining items in various ways may reduce the user's insight and cause a different meaning to be attached to the message. We measure disorder, dispersion or centralization, in entropy terms, using Shannon's formula. Consider an organization containing three levels of operations: a single supreme decision-maker; four second-level controllers and four third-level controllers. Suppose half the organizational decisions are made by the single supreme decision-maker. The remaining decisions are distributed as one-quarter to the second level and one-quarter to the third level. In the second and third levels each of the controllers share equally in the decisions. The entropy of the organization, that is, the degree of centralization in decision-making turns out to be approximately equal to a single-level organization, with six managers sharing equally in the decision-making process.

---

1. Lev, B., The aggregation problem in financial statements: an informational approach, J. Accounting Res., Vol. 8, 1968, 247-61.
2. Lev, B., The informational approach to aggregation in financial statements, J. Accounting Res., Vol. 8, 1970, 78-94.
3. Theil, H., On the use of information theory concepts in the analysis of financial statements, Management Science, Vol. 15, 1969, 459-80.

Davis[1] and Lisiman[2] suggested money as the analog of economic entropy, a concept transcending the Leontief static input-output equations (economic processes completely described by the flow of commodities into and out of the system).[3] Georgescu-Roegen[4] recommended some biological homologies to account for changes with time that Leontief ignored. The economic process is entropic; it neither creates nor consumes matter or energy but only transforms low-entropy systems to higher levels. Money constitutes the economic equivalent of low entropy[5,6]; gold is the social equivalent of biological energy.[6] We seek a conversion factor to find the entropy equivalent of economic value. Entropy changes in closed chemical systems have been traced for about one hundred and twenty years; for open systems it is ninety years. Extension of the open system analysis into situations far from equilibrium earned Prigogine the 1977 Nobel Prize in chemistry. Even before this, entropy and biological processes were linked[7]; later entropy and business activity were joined.[8] Perhaps the earliest work in irreversible thermodynamics was Thompson's examination of steady state open systems[9]: the creation and maintenance of a concentration difference across a film of liquid with a temperature difference. The heat flow caused the concentration gradient; the concentration gradient implied order (a higher order than before and less

---

1. Davis, H.T., The theory of econometrics, Bloomington, Indiana U. Press, 1941, 1971-6.
2. Lisiman, J.H.C., Econometrics and thermodynamics: A remark on Davis' theory of budgets, Econometrica, XVII, 1949, 59-62.
3. Leontief, W.W., The structure of the American economy: 1919-1939, New York, 1951.
4. Georgescu-Roegen, N., The entropy law and economic processes, Harvard U. Press, Cambridge, Mass., 1971.
5. Helm, G., Die lehre von der energie, Leipzig, 1887.
6. Winiarsk, L., Essai sue le mechanique sociale: L'energie sociale et ses mensurations, Part II, Revue Philosophique, XLIX, 1900, 265, 287.
7. Lotka, A., Elements of physical biology, Williams and Wilkins, Baltimore, 1925.
8. Myers, S., V. Flowers, A framework for measuring human assets, California Management Review, 1974, 516.
9. Denbigh, K.G., The thermodynamics of the steady-state, Wiley, London, 1958.

entropy). All caused by the heat flow. Onsager too won a Nobel Prize for his thermodynamic work on irreversible processes[1] not far from equilibrium, driven by modest forces. Prigogine and his coworkers went beyond Onsager and developed theories for the appearance of new structures far from equilibrium[2], beginning with the decomposition of the entropy production term into two parts: from the internal irreversible reactions and the interactions of system and environment.[3] Social organizations as diverse as informal friendships and cultures have definable conditions of order and efficiency just as surely as do steam engines. Three basic flow categories have been identified which cross corporate boundaries[4]: matter, energy and information. Specific flows into the system include, among others, raw materials, supplies, equipment, services, work by employees, information and capital, usually expressed in monetary not entropy terms. The flows out of a manufacturing operation are products, by-products, wastes, information and dividends. There are also pressures from the environment: government regulations and actions of competitors. Internal processes include the aging of employees and equipment, generation of novel information, changes in organizational structure and conflicts among employees. The search for a relationship between value and entropy began around 1880[5,6] when money became "sociobiological energy", a simplistic approach to an esoteric question. Suppose we are to boil water using alternatively, wood, natural gas and coal as the fuel. The entropy change of the water, in going from liquid water to steam is

---

1. Myers, S., V. Flowers, op. cited.
2. Prigogine, I., Introduction to the thermodynamics of irreversible processes, C.C. Thomas, Springfield, Illinois, 1955.
3. Georgian, J., The MKS temperature scale, J. Chem. Eng., Vol. 43, 1966, 414.
4. Iberall, M., Social systems and the dissipative model, General Systems Yearbook, Vol. XIX, 1974, 201.
5. Gurevitch, K., Geographical differentiation and its measures in a discrete system, Soviet Geography, Vol. 10, 1969, 387-412.
6. Shock, N., et. al., Age differences in the water content of the body related to basal oxygen consumption in males, J. Gerontology, Vol. 18, 1963, 1.

the same if we begin at the same temperature and pressure and end similarly for each of the three different burning processes. But the cost of the product, steam, depends on which fuel is used and hence the entropy-money conversion cost is not fixed. Ostwald[1] proposed that economic value depends only on the energy stored and available in the wood, natural gas or coal but it should be pointed out that the efficiency of the burning process is also important. (The value of the steam may depend on whether the wood is burned in an open fire or in a controlled draft furnace.) Entropy changes can be calculated for: water to ice transformations; carbon dioxide gas to solid dry ice changes; the graphite-diamond correspondence and helium gas-helium liquid phase inversions. Depending on the energy, equipment and labor cost we can produce empirical correlations to describe an entropy-money conversion factor.[2] If these factors were readily available, we could make an entropy balance around a corporate open system and establish its entropy exchange with the environment. Since the late 1940's entropy calculations using Shannon's formula have analyzed the dispersion of decision-making in the business world, between groups and within groups in a hierarchical organization.[3] For example, consider a hypothetical soap market consisting of three competitors, A, B, and C, each selling products, 1, 2 and 3. Suppose the total market share for company A, B, and C is PA, PB and PC; each product share is P1, P2, and P3. Let the total market for companies A, B, and C be 18 units. We might get the following fictive numbers:

---

1. Ostwald, W., Die Energie, 1908, 1964.
2. Davis, M.G., A quantitative application of entropy production analysis for small profit-seeking organizations, M.S. Thesis, U. of Cincinnati, Cincinnati, Ohio 1978.
3. Philippatos, G.C., N. Gressis, Conditions of equilibrium among E-V, SSD and E-H portfolio selection criteria: the case for uniform, normal and lognormal distributions; Management Science, Vol. 21, 1975, 617-25.

Company A	Company B	Company C
$PA = \frac{5}{18}$	$PB = \frac{5}{18}$	$PC = \frac{8}{18}$
$P1 = \frac{1}{18}$	$P1 = \frac{3}{18}$	$P1 = \frac{3}{18}$
$P2 = \frac{3}{18}$	$P2 = \frac{1}{18}$	$P3 = \frac{3}{18}$
$P3 = \frac{1}{18}$	$P3 = \frac{1}{18}$	$P3 = \frac{2}{18}$

In the business world of marketing, there are two basic assumptions made: (1) a firm's market share is assumed to represent the probability that a customer will purchase a product at random and (2) those same probabilities represent a customer's freedom of choice.[1] Using our example, P1 = 18/18 = 1.0 would signify no freedom of choice, for one product has captured the entire market (a monopolistic situation); Shannon's formula would yield an informational entropy value of zero. In marketing, entropy serves to ascertain the degree of uncertainty in the market—which is to say that it reflects the degree of competition among firms. Higher entropy values are synonymous with a healthy level of competition (a more disorganized market with competition evenly distributed).

Hahn[2] attempted to establish a relationship between the usual corporate performance indicators such as profits, sales, etc. and informational entropy. The goal was to correlate fiscal performance with internal hierarchical structure (the table of organization). Corporate structure was written as a coven of blocks, such as those for the President, and the Vice President for Sales. Each block was characterized by a power factor containing two parameters: (1) the fraction of the total corporate budget controlled and (2) the hierarchial level below the President (where the top rung is 1, Vice Presidents are 2, etc.). Thus the measure of power each

---
1. Horwitz, A.R., I. Horwitz, Entropy, markov processes and competition in the brewing industry, Industrial Economics, Vol. 16, 1968, 196-211.
2. Hahn, J.C., An application of informational entropy concepts to profit-seeking organizations, M.S. Thesis, U. of Cincinnati, Cincinnati, Ohio 1979.

organizational block carries is directly related to its budgetary responsibility and inversely proportional to the distance from the ultimate decision-maker, the President. Changes in fiscal performance were mapped along with entropies calculated by Shannon's formula (the power factor represented the decision-making frequency). This preliminary study of Hahn's suggests that an optimum structural configuration may exist, where performance and productivity can be maximized within an organization by establishing which internal structure is most conducive for optimum information flow. Shannon's formula is a useful tool here for deriving entropy data [1-5] because: (1) maximum entropy seems to correlate well with the most highly disordered state; (2) increasing the number of hierarchical blocks raises the organizational entropy; (3) higher entropy values are synonymous with greater competition and (4) we can glean from entropy a measure of concentration and dispersion. An inefficient and disorganized company should evidence high entropy and high operating expenses. For the jejune company there will probably be a jump in profits as size and structure increase—up to the point where size and structure begin to work against an efficient operation. There can be, with some structures, too little informational entropy (the capacity to transmit information) where insufficient capacity to transmit information means too much information is being stored and not used.[6] This excess of stored information (calculated from Shannon's formula) could likely garble the lines of communication between the various departments of a corporation, manifested by tedious administrative and clerical detail as well as excessive interdepartmental

---

1. Horowitz, I., Employment concentration in the common market: an entropy approach, J. Roy. Statist. Soc., vol. 133, 1970, 463-75.
2. Philippatos, G.C., N. Gressis, op. cited.
3. Horwitz, A.R., I. Horowitz, op. cited, 196-211.
4. Thiel, H., Economics and information theory, Chicago, Rand-McNally, 1967.
5. Finkelstein, M.O., R.M. Friedberg, The application of an entropy of concentration to the Clayton Act, Yale Law Journal, vol. 76, 1967, 677-717.
6. Gatlin, op. cited.

formality and reserve The result could be a hierarchy so complex and rigid that the system's ability to disseminate information quickly to its components and to respond with flexibility in the face of change is seriously undermined. (Another factor working to efface flexibility in economic systems is inflation.[1] It heightens the uncertainty surrounding economic transactions, attenuates the links between effect and reward, increases the role of luck in success, decreases the influence of hard work and diminishes the legitimacy of market-determined rewards. The major debilitating influence of inflation is the debauchment of the currency and the threatening of the free enterprise economic system.[2] Those who the system brings windfalls become profiteers who are the objects of the hatred of the bourgeoise, whom inflation has impoverished. There may be no subtler, no surer means of overturning the existing basis of society than to traduce the currency.)

Living systems are born, mature, senesce and die, all performing their little dance of life within a finite time frame. It is easy to plot their course for we know there is a beginning, a middle and an end. For so-called inanimate systems such as corporations, countries and civilizations, it is not as simple a matter to identify the opening event, birth, or the denouement, death, with such clarity. What of mergers? How to account for human intercedence, which alters the course of history? Who can say that a country has died when it is conquered? Do civilizations really expire? Toynbee[3] searched for the forces which bring a civilization to birth: "I first try race and then environment and I find both of these explanations unsatisfying because they assume that living beings are subject to inexorable laws of Nature ... I find that although a strong stimulus is needed to bring a civilization into existence, the challenge (and then response) must not be so severe as to stifle creativity".

---

1. Higgs, R., Inflation and the destruction of the free marked economy, The Intercollegiate Review, 1979, 657-76.
2. Keynes, J.M., The Economic consequences of the peace, New York, Harcourt, Brace and Howe, 1920, 235-6.
3. Toynbee, A., A study of history, Oxford U. Press, 1972, 73.

What is it that drives us to new structures? Is it creativity, challenge and response, the stimulus of different environments (terrain), the stimulus of penalizations such as religious discrimination? A nascent civilization has surmounted the first and highest hurdle but will it then go from strength to strength? And for how long? A society continues to grow, it seems, when successful response to a challenge provokes a fresh challenge to be met, converting a single action into a series of movements. The growth of a society can be measured in terms of its increasing power of self-determination; the future lies in the hands of the creative minority. A civilization that attempts some extraordinary tour de force may find itself not defeated outright, but arrested in a state of immobility, its energies absorbed in meeting the single great challenge. The Central Asian Nomads were condemned to this fate: they successfully mastered the problem of adaptation to the harsh exigencies of life on the steppes, but in doing so they became the slaves of their environment, unable to make any fresh creative advances.[1] The movement of challenge-and-response becomes a self-sustaining series if each successful response provokes a disequilibrium, requiring new creative adjustment. Prometheus, after defying a tyrannical Zeus by bringing the forbidden power of fire to Man, next wins the right for perpetual development. Society is a network of relations, the interaction of two or more agents. A society is the medium of communication through which humans interact. Growth is assured through integration to differentiation to reintegration and thence to redifferentiation. The process by which growth of civilizations is sustained is inherently risky: the creative leadership of a society has to carry along the uncreative mass. The ultimate failure of creativity seems to stem from its successes, whereby we seem to become lazy or self-satisfied or conceited. These numinous successes inspire others to follow but often creates a requirement for dull obedience, such as soldiers in an

---

1. Toynbee, A., op. cited, 128.

army. In some civilizations, an army on becoming demoralized degenerates into rebellion.

Spengler[1] argues that a civilization is comparable to an organism, subjected to the same processes of childhood, youth, maturity and old age as a human being or any other living thing. He claims every civilization, every archaic age, every rise and downfall has a definite time frame which is always the same and which always recurs.[2] Plato[3] refers to a society with an idealized constitution that is therefore not easily thrown out of equilibrium—but will eventually disintegrate as is everything else foredoomed this way. The breakdown is connected with the periodic rhythm of life—in animals, the vegetable kingdom and the so-called inanimate world. Or do you subscribe to the belief that civilizations succeed one another by a natural law of the cosmos, in a perpetually recurrent cycle of alternating births and deaths.[4]

Do you accept the premise that civilizations have met their death not from the assault of external and uncontrollable forces but by their own hands? We become complacent; we lose the Promethean elan of the unstable equilibrium in which custom and mimesis are never allowed to become entrenched. The arrested societies in history (the Ottoman Turks, the Spartans, the Eurasian Nomadic society) have achieved so close an adaptation to their environment that they become the scriven, assuming its color and rhythm instead of impressing upon the environment their own prosody. The forces acting upon the arrested society demand so much of their energies simply to maintain the position already attained; there is nothing left for reconnoitering the course ahead. The nemesis of creativity in a civilization is the idolization of an ephemeral self or institution. Toynbee illustrates this point[5]: "A classic case in which

---
1. Spengler, O., Der untergang des abendlander, Vienna and Leipzig, Wilhelm Braunmuller, 1918, I, 152-3.
2. Spengler, O., op. cited, 160-1.
3. Plato, Respublica, 546 A-B.
4. Eliade, M., Le mythe de l'eternal retour, Paris, Gallimand, 1949.
5. Toynbee, A., op. cited, 180.

the idolization of an institution brought down an entire civilization was the infatuation of Orthodox Christendom with a ghost of the Roman Empire, an ancient institution which had fulfilled its historical function and completed its natural term of life before Orthodox Christian Society made its attempt to resuscitate it. In Orthodox Christendom from the eighth century onwards the loyalty which should have been reserved for the Orthodox Christian Society as a whole was restricted to a single institution—the East Roman Empire. From the tenth century onwards, the expanding Orthodox Christendom had embraced the Bulgars as well as the Greeks within the Orthodox Christendom fold; from 927 the Orthodox idolaters were divided between one parochial Empire in Constantinople and another at Preslav. Since both Empires claimed an ecumenical jurisdiction by divine right, a life-and-death struggle between them was inevitable; with the idolater's house divided against itself, it was no wonder that it could not stand".[1] Breakdowns of civilizations may not be inevitable and perhaps not irretrievable, but in the process of disintegration, if allowed to fester, they show some similarities with the myriad of social systems. The masses became estranged from their leaders, who then try to cling to their positions by using force as a substitute for their evanescent power of attraction. A dying society molders in a climate of violence, seen by the victors as a cataclysm in which the forces of evil are destroyed and a new age of peace inaugurated. In a disintegrating society, the "internal proleteriat", the spiritually dispossessed, are the catalysts for regeneration. The "external proleteriat" borrows and exploits the culture of its civilized neighbor. Demoralized by their failures, the people of a disintegrating society resort to parodies of the creative inspiration they seem to have lost. The cults which arise are generally barren and in general represent an attempted escape from an intolerable world. In passing from the breakdown of a civilization to its disintegration, we should not readily assume that this sequence is

---
1. Toynbee, A., op. cited, 195.

automatic and unalterable—that once a civilization has broken down it must inevitably drive towards disintegration and dissolution. Although this was the pattern of the Hellenic Civilization, it is not necessarily true for all civilizations.[1] The Egyptian Society, in spite of its having broken down before the end of the third millennium B.C., refused to disappear and actually succeeded in surviving for another 2500 years—a span of time that was perhaps nearly three times as long as the longevity of its birth, growth and first breakdown. It's survival was however, bought at a price, for this society during the second eon of existence was in seeming suspended animation; it survived by becoming calcified. During the growth process, a challenge is only met once. For so long as growth is being maintained, each challenge is successfully overcome and the civilization moves on. By contrast, in the disintegration of civilizations, the perpetual variety and versatility which are hallmarks of growth yield a noisome uniformity and uninventiveness. After the failure to meet the challenges, the old unanswered challenges reappear wraithlike to present themselves more insistently and in even more virulent form until at last they dominate and obsess and overwhelm the society. Thus the disintegration of a civilization, like its growth is a cumulative and continuous process. In essence, the loss of harmony between previously coexisting elements in a society leads ineluctably to social discord. There are vertical schisms among geographically segregated communities and horizontal schisms operating on geographically intermingled but successfully segregated classes.[2] The horizontal schism of a society along lines of class appears at the moment of breakdown, a distinctive benchmark, absent during the growth phase (using the Hellenic civilization as our paradigm[3]). The conjoining social mechanisms which drove the French Revolution were diagnosed by **Saint-Simon**.[4] The disintegration

---
1. Toynbee, A., op. cited, 59.
2. Toynbee, A., op. cited, Part I, Chapter 7.
3. Toynbee, A., op. cited, 56.
4. Bzard, A., Exposition de la doctrine saint simonienne, in Oeuvres de saint-simon et d'enfantin, Paris, Leroux, 1877, XLI, 171-4.

began when status was questioned and hostile fragments arose. The ruthless pursuit of incompatible class interests shatters the social pyramid and creates new structures of oppression. The external proleteriat, like the internal proleteriat, creates itself by an act of secession from the dominant minority of a civilization that has broken down. The internal proleteriat continues to live intermingled geographically with the dominant minority from which it has become divided by a moral gulf; the external proleteriat is not only alienated from the dominant minority emotionally but also physically, by a frontier which can be traced on a map. In a growing civilization the creative minority can exercise its powers of attraction upon neighbors beyond its borders as well as upon the internal community (as witness the adoption of the Syrian alphabet in Manchuria, or the reflection of Hellenic aesthetic styles in the coins of Celtic Britain and in the statuary of Northern India[1]). The diddling of a disintegrating society emboldens its neighbors, who now become a menace: a symptom of the malaise of the Hellenic Civilization was the civil war of 431-401 B.C. and the invasion of Macedonia by a Thracian horde, the end of the voluntary Hellenization of Thrace. A weakened Roman Empire from the fourth to the sixth century was under continual attack on its northern front by successive waves of Huns, Avars, Teutons and Slavs, piling up against each other and eventually overrunning the whole of Rome's Empire in the West.

When a society is disintegrating, the dominant minority tries to preserve its threatened power by uniting the warring nations (the external proleteriat) into a universal state or empire, a seemingly single civilization. The creation of a universal state checks the headlong decline of a disintegrating civilization; such states are endorsed eagerly by those who believe their empire is destined to be as immortal as the gods who have ordained it. This conviction is sustained by the vainglorious assertion that their universal state will embrace the whole world, leaving of course no external force to threaten it.

---

1. Toynbee, A., op, cited, 234.

This misplaced confidence in immortality and universality is exemplified by the Roman Empire. The prestige of universal states may outlive their reality, even after the power has evaporated. (In India, the Emperor Akbas II in 1803 was the puppet of British masters. He performed the empty ritual of receiving representatives of the British India Company, balm for him and a ploy which hid the reality of total control by the British.[1]) Universal states unify one civilization, but also embrace portions of alien societies. The peoples of the Russian Empire, from Armenia to Lapland and from the Ukraine to Siberia show the panoramic extent of the Russian universal state in the eighteenth century. For the rulers of universal states a network of communications is an indispensable instrument of military and political control; the most famous road system is probably that of the Roman Empire, the universal state of the Hellenic world. In a universal state the capital city derives enormous prestige from its status as the seat of government. The degree of efficiency attained by imperial administration varied considerably among universal states. In Rome and in British India the commercial middle class was gradually insinuated into the administration; British administration in India until the end of the eighteenth century was in the hands of the East India Company's commercial officers. Universal states are essentially negative institutions; they arise after, not before, the breakdown of the civilization to which they purport to bring political unity. They are the products of dominant minorities: the once creative minorities that lost their Promethean power. They are systems of social disintegration. Universal states seem to be possessed by an almost demonic craving for life; their citizens believe passionately in the immortality of their country or institution. Livy[2] (59 B.C.—17 A.D.) writing of the Roman Empire said, "the city founded to endure forever at the instance of the Gods". However long the life of a universal state may be drawn out, it has always proved to

---

1. Toynbee, A., op cited, 257-265.
2. Toynbee, A., op. cited, 267.

be the last phase of a society before its extinction. It's goal is the achievement of immortality, a vain effort to thwart the economy of Nature. There is a perpetual need for raw material to provide for the growth of later ages. Life is given to none of us in perpetuity.[1]

Most empires, the Sinic, the Roman and the East Roman Empire have been universal only in that they laid claim to worldwide dominion. Of all the universal states cited by Toynbee, only two—China and Russia—are still in existence today. These states now claim only to be the leading political vehicle of an ideology they proclaim as the sole true faith for all the world. Toynbee posited the likelihood that the world states of the future will begin by being a voluntary political association in which the cultural elements of a number of living civilizations will continue to assert themselves.[2] The west has continued its cultural invasion of the other living civilizations of the world for the past five hundred years but now we are learning the dolorous lesson not to automatically assume that the values and goals of our own civilization will be permanently dominant. We cannot be sure that new civilizations will not emerge in the future or that those which at present seem to be submerged will not be revivified. Most of the universal states that have united civilizations politically have subsumed parts of other civilizations and their own barbarians or dissenters. The founders of universal states have recognized and tolerated cultural, linguistic and religious diversity: the Achaemenian Empire's policy of religious toleration, for example.[3] We long for a world united in peace and freedom, recognizing that the bitter experience of war and anarchy moves us towards a utopian salvation, the unification of rival parochial polities. Sometimes, as in the past, this dream has resulted in tyranny and even when it did not, the pressures for unification and the formation of a universal state presaged the eventual downfall of a society. Civilizations are brought to grief by

---

1. Lucretius, De Rerum Natura, III, 964-5, 967-71.
2. Toynbee, A., op. cited, 318.
3. Toynbee, A., op, cited, 318.

their own faults and failures, not always by external agencies. A society in the process of dissolution is usually overrun and finally liquidated by so-called barbarians from beyond its frontiers, the pressure built up by frontiers which have become seemingly impermeable. The barbarians are the brooms which sweep the historical stage clear of the debris of a dead civilization, much as the phagocytes of our bodies perform their tasks for us. The weakened civilization, temporarily reconstituted in a universal state surrounds itself with rigid political frontiers which repel the attractive forces of the barbarians. Not able to imitate the culture and art of the universal state, frustrated, the barbarians attack. The fluid zone of contact between the universal state and the adjacent barbarians has become frozen into a seemingly impenetrable military frontier: neighbors become enemies and cultural exchanges cease. Hadrian's Wall was visible evidence of the Roman Empire's attempt to insulate itself from the barbarian tribes of northern Britain and to protect against invasion.[1] China's Great Wall, consolidated by the Ch'in dynasty in the third century, B.C., is tangible evidence of an embattled civilization's attempt to establish rigid lines of defense against outer barbarians. Some embattled civilizations that died, according to Toynbee[2] are:

Eighteenth Century B.C.	The Egyptian Middle Kingdom was destroyed by Hyksos invaders.
Third Century B.C.–Second Century A.D.	Mauryan Empire broken up after the death of Acoka, succumbing to Bactrian Greek Invaders led by Demetrius at the beginning of the second century.
Fourth and Fifth Century A.D.	The Gupta dynasty reestablished the unity that had been lost with the disintegration of Mauryan India. The Gupta Empire declined under the impact of Hun and Gurjara invasion.

---

1. Toynbee, A., op. cited, 354.
2. Toynbee, A., op. cited, 500.

Fourth and Fifth Century B.C.	The Archaemenian Empire united the Syriac and Iranian Worlds in one universal state. East and West were linked by the Scythian Trail trade route across the steppes occupied by pastoral Nomad barbarians. The civilizations at the extreme east and west of the old worlds were in a phase of political disunity at the time. It dissolved by the second century.
First and Second Century A.D.	The two great universal states of the Old World, the Roman and Han Empires were kept from direct contact by the Parthian Arsacid and Kushan States, both founded by barbarian Nomads. A cordon of barbarian people was pressing upon the northern frontiers of all Empires.
Eleventh and Twelfth Century A.D.	The breakup of the Arab and Chinese universal states left a mosaic of smaller states. The Holy Roman Empire was merely the largest of these.
Thirteenth and Fourteenth Century A.D.	The conquests of the Mongols united almost the entire Eurasian land-mass in one universal state. Only two Muslim states, one in India and the other in Syria and Egypt retained their independence.

Chapter 19
A Kid's View of Death

Puff will die soon, perhaps in five years. Michael, will you understand why a dog also dies? Will you accept the death of this loving animal who has been our companion, who has protected us, been our playmate and even our teacher? How will Puff die? Will she be hit by an automobile and have the life crushed from her? Will she be gored by yet another german shephard as happened in the past and will our frantic rush to the hospital be unsuccessful next time? Or will she just get old and infirmed, lose her vitality and die quietly? Will you accept the fact that she will in old age look as youthful as when she was younger, thus destroying one of your bases for judging who is to die? Michael, you do not as yet acknowledge that dead is the same as being killed. You kill often, with your imaginary guns and bullets and bows and arrows and karate chops. Regularly you slash off heads of those who are in mock battle against you. You kill them but they are not dead and you are able to fight them again the next day. So far, Michael, you cannot conceive of the finality of death. Dead is like being killed, Michael, and soon, too soon, you shall see this. I expect your education will rapidly resolve this dichotomy and I mourn for your loss of innocence.

Chapter 20

Do You Know Me, Michael?

Michael, your presence is such an important part of my life. I ponder the very serious question: Would I give up my life for yours? Where the ultimate decision is demanded, is it I or you who will live? Would I sacrifice my life so that yours could continue? Having lived some decades and seen happiness and pain, I am at a station in life which is the culmination of my life's ambitions, with most of my conscious goals accomplished. I am quite ready to step down, out of the game if it will keep you in it. I believe great things are done in this world not in isolated steps, but rather by a continuum of small progressions. It's becoming your turn. I can only refine and redefine my activities, do little adjustments here and there, but for you, the great discoveries are yet to come.

Who am I? Do you sense that I believe in moderation, in a balanced approach to things, that we should be able to understand all points of view, but not tolerate pompous asses? Do you understand my sense of universality, within our world and beyond, for all living things? Is it clear that I cannot accept the canard that Americans are inherently better human beings than others, that one religion has a direct pipeline to God and not the others? Do you discern how important this has become for me, that the aging process needs to be studied, that old people need to be more fully understood and cared for if they are in need? And that we must treat them with the dignity they have earned. Do you know me, Michael?

Love,
Daddy

Chapter 21

The Challenge: The Search For Unifying Principles

In this survey of aging systems, I have sought homologous principles upon which to tether an analysis. Whether we examine living systems or the so-called inanimate corporation, cities or civilizations, it seems apparent that the concept of entropy cannot be ignored. For innately bound to entropy are the key phrases, the code words we need to apply to these complex, sometimes inchoate, othertimes baroque systems: structure; energy; information flow; stability; fluctuations; dissipation and evolution. We require a means for measuring the order and control of the life process within us, to calculate our energy levels and resiliency in meeting the stresses of life. By entropy calculations we ought to be able to establish our state of disorder and how rapidly we are descending towards death. Entropy as the measure of disorder can provide the direction of life. And do we die when the entropy numbers suggest a low point in our rate of living, the asymptotic approach to the state where evolution ceases and the energy to drive us onward is lacking? Stasis and death, the final denouement?

The corporation at first blush seems different but is it really so divergent? True, while we living systems do die—must die—the corporations escape. They die in a way by going bankrupt or merging. Yet rejuvenation is always possible as the management team charts a new course. We can examine flows into and out of the corporate system and assign entropy values to these. Surely the internal structure can be fleshed out and appropriate informational entropies calculated with Shannon's formula. And will this entropy balance on this consumate example of an open system yield a rate of living and entropy production which can be correlated with profits and products? Is there a collateral exchange between entropy production, information flow, productivity and profits? Ask the Chrysler Corporation. We can chart a corporation's evolution from nascence, to maturity to senescence and even death for the bankrupt and ask to what extent is it reversible.

The challenge for us is to examine the structure of our systems and seek a unified theory within which can be subsumed life and death, the rise and fall, of living organisms, corporations, cities and civilizations. In so doing we shall treat them as open systems, exchanging mass, energy and information with their surroundings yet concomitantly engaging in the internal irreversibilities we have previously mentioned. The approach therefore, is to define entropy generation terms for both the internal and external operations. For living systems this seems straightforward. Air in and out during breathing can be characterized according to its entropy content. Our bodily functions have been shown to translate into entropy production by way of the basal metabolic rate. The wear and tear (rate of living) theory of aging provides guidance on how to establish limits on lifespan. For corporations we can do the same. The flows across boundaries, be they raw materials, information, energy, products, wastes, etc. may be expressed in entropy units by appropriate money-entropy or information-entropy conversion factors. The internal structure can be partitioned according to function, budget and distance from the fountainhead. Using Shannon's formula, informational entropy content can be established and added to the net entropy exchanged across the boundaries. A chronological history of the corporation may then be constructed detailing entropy production and function versus age. How shall we define the juvenile state? Maturity? Senility? How are the stability criteria of Prigogine to be applied? Can we define the fluctuations which will force the corporation to new structures? Is it a self-organizing system driven to new forms by business pressures? And can we do the same for cities and civilizations, alive, moribund or dead? This is our challenge. What is your response?